Been There. Done That. Finally Getting it Right. Developing Authentic Individual Education Plans for Students with Autism

Lessons from a Mother and Teacher

ISBN 978-0-9813388-0-4

Published by Autism Aspirations, Peterborough, Ontario
Canada

www.autismaspirations.com

To my students,

I dedicate this book to all my students with autism -you have been so patient with me as I continue to learn from you. I did not choose this journey and yet, my life is so rich and rewarding because each of you has journeyed with me and taught me more than I can ever teach you. I love each and every one of you.

To my family,

Karli, Kieran and Kaiya, each of you have lived with me being 'present but not really there' as the pages of this book unfolded. Thank you for reminding me to get my head out of the book! I love each of you beyond words; you give me purpose and joy. You are deeply loved and appreciated.

Kieran, you allow me to open your life and experiences up to the readers so that others may find hope and reassurance. You are a gift to our family and to the world. We love you.

My husband, Ivars, you are my partner and my best friend. You encourage me to be all that I can be and together we have made a difference. I love you.

Jenn
(aka: Mrs. K., and Mom)

Who is Jennifer Krumins?

Each child's birth changes the face of the world and brings with it new hope and a fresh beginning. Never could I have imagined what gifts my children would bring to my life: passion, clarity, and purpose. But life also has a way of delivering the greatest gifts wrapped in the disguise of grief. When our second child was diagnosed with severe autism our life as we knew it (and planned it) changed dramatically.

Our own son and the students that I have had the privilege of teaching have made me take a hard look at what I value and what I believe about purpose and fulfillment in life. They have collectively taught me that getting ahead doesn't bring happiness but looking into the eyes of a child that finally conquers a skill...now that is pure joy! My kids have taught me to really tune into my senses; truly feel the sun on my skin and the smell of a spring day. My kids have taught me to slow down and really look at even the most insignificant things in life and see their glory. I have learned that our productivity doesn't make us loveable; we already are. Our purpose in life isn't about financial gain and material prosperity; it is about accepting ourselves and being at peace with who we are; living our lives for the sake of bringing some peace and happiness to others. My kids with autism have taught me more than I could hope to teach them.

Raising a child with autism has taught my husband of 22 years and me the most important lessons in life: present difficulties are defined by our attitudes far more than by the challenging circumstances; stay optimistic, build relationships whenever possible and rely on your faith.

Riding the tidal wave of autism is a voyage of a life time but the rewards are profound and immeasurable. This is not to diminish in any way the heart -wrenching, exhaustive and heartbreaking nature of autism but we refused to look at it that way. Even through the tears, we knew that our son was here to teach us something. Individuals with autism have gifts that they bring to the world. Sadly, the world doesn't always recognize these treasures.

My husband and I have 3 children: two daughters aged 20 and 12 and our son who is 18 years old. Teaching in Ontario, Canada for 23 years has equipped me with vast experience in all kinds of learning differences and challenging learning difficulties. But none would compare with teaching my own son both in the general classroom (for two years) and in private therapy at home. It was these experiences that both drained me emotionally and inspired me professionally. Being the teacher and the mom brought me face to face with my own teaching philosophy and my teaching practices. Living on both sides of a child's education taught me many lessons in advocacy. The critical role of building relationships, compromise and empathy became crystal clear as I sat in both the teacher and parent role.

I earned Masters of Education in Human Development and Applied Psychology at the Ontario Institute for Studies in Education. Raising a son with autism motivated me to obtain a Special Education Specialist and to train extensively at Queen's University in Kingston, Ontario and the Geneva Centre for Autism in Toronto, Ontario. I had the privilege of working in a private therapy program for my son under the guidance and direction of the Behaviour Institute in Hamilton, Ontario. But most importantly, I have been privileged to work with students with autism that have given me the best education imaginable.

I have been blessed with a family and a career that have enriched my life and made me who I am today. I want to share what I have learned and do my part to open the doors for students that have autism, their teachers and their parents. I want to facilitate collaboration, teamwork and mutual understanding in the education of our children. It is my belief that Autism has the potential to create more compassionate communities and families if we accept the challenge of working together to recognize the strengths, develop weaknesses and celebrate the diversity of autistic minds.

Welcome to the journey! You are not alone. ☺

Jenn

Table of Contents

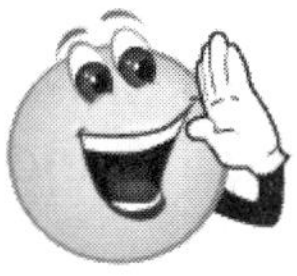

Important: Read This First

It's only fair that I be honest right from the start. I don't enjoy creating individual education plans. I have a hard time deciding what goals to choose, especially when a student's needs are high. I want to do it all and be all I can for the student who needs me most. I hate how scripted and hemmed in I feel by IEPs - always striving to be clear and concise while incorporating the correct terminology and prescribed components. Frustration grips me at times when I am trying to transform ideas into meaningful SMART goals. Instinct about what I really want for a student clashes with the question of how I can put that knowledge into a well written goal and subsequent objectives. I especially hate trying to decide how I will measure the goal! I find writing individual education plans tiring and mind bending at times.

You might think that having researched IEPs for years, written books and consulted in the development of them, I would hold some perverse pleasure in the documents. No, quite the opposite; the more I learn, the more I confound my own ability to create a simple and authentic product. Lurking in the shadows of my awareness is the suspicion that no one will really even look at the IEP when it is complete. Does anyone actually pore over it and integrate its ideas into daily practice? I cringe considering the answer.

Despite my feelings, I must concede that the core of my beliefs as an educator center on individualizing education based on the unique qualities of each student. Long ago, the concept of cookie cutter teaching was replaced by reality. In addition, when I strip away all the reasons I entered the profession: my love for talking and for kids, the weird excitement I feel when I am in a teacher supply store, the challenge of making tough concepts understandable and - the holidays, I am left with something big inside of me. Something that often gets obscured by the craziness of the daily demands.

In the essence of who I am there lies an unchanging, profound desire to make someone feel good about themselves. Twenty some years of teaching has not changed this deep drive within me. There is simply no better feeling in the world than to be a part of facilitating growth in an individual of any age. Even the crappiest of days can be transformed by one small moment when a student looks into my eyes and I witness the unmistakable glow that proclaims, "I get it!" This declaration reflects the deeper and unspoken thrill of the words, "I *am* smart!"

So what does this have to do with an individual education plan? Everything. An IEP will only be as valuable to the degree that it reflects a genuine desire to help a child be his/her best self. Let's be clear, and maybe a little harsh: if you are going to view the IEP as a formal hoop completed with as little time, energy and enthusiasm as possible, in order to appease some external force, then I suggest the final product will indeed be quite uninspiring. It will be done. You will have fulfilled your duty. But, you will have missed an opportunity to transcend the drudgery.

An individual education plan gives us an occasion to use the gifts that brought us to a career in education: creating a vision for another person's life, thinking through the steps of getting there, and finally, crafting activities and strategies to facilitate growth towards the vision. Without meaning to diminish our role as teachers, many students will have the intellect and skills to achieve their goals with minimal direct intervention from us. But, as you are well aware, there are students who need our skills, our creativity and our compassion more than others in order to grow towards their potential.

IEPs can make a difference when they are viewed with a growth mindset: the core belief that intelligence and abilities can be developed (Dweck, 2007). Personal growth in ourselves and in our students is not only possible but expected. When we allow ourselves to dream with and for the child, we create far more than a legal document, but a roadmap of the best travel plans we can conceive. And we begin the journey one small step at a time.

When we allow ourselves to dream with and for the child, we create far more than a legal document, but a roadmap of the best travel plans we can conceive.

The fact that you have chosen to read this book tells me that you and I share a passion for educating children and facilitating the growth of human potential. If by chance you were coerced into reading this, I am sorry. It will not be a gripping, page turner. But, if you can keep an open mind and hold a student you care about in your mind's eye, it just may help you to grow as an educator. My hope is that somehow through reading this book you will feel less alone, more competent and empowered to be the best educator you can be.

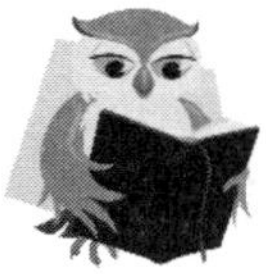

We should not live in the clouds, on a superficial level. We should dedicate ourselves to understanding our brothers and sisters.

Mother Teresa

Welcome to a New School Year!

It's the end of summer. For parents, students and teachers alike, this month brings with it the excitement of a new year and a fresh start as well as the anxiety and concern of the unknown. Parents may question: Who will be the teacher? Will he know and understand autism? Will my thoughts and concerns be heard and valued? Students may wonder: Will the teacher like me? Will I be able to succeed? And teachers may worry: Will I be able to reach this child? Will I have the support of the parent? Will I have a team to help me or will I be on my own? The angst of a new year is felt by everyone involved and sleepless nights are common as summer winds down!

But, on the other hand, there is a renewed hope for a new year. The success of a new year has everything to do with how each person involved approaches it. Parents, teachers and professionals have a fresh chance to embrace a team mentality. Together the team can raise the child to new heights when each person adopts a 'growth mindset' both for the student and the adults working for the student.

The road on this journey will be challenging: assumptions, strong emotions and miscommunications are to be expected. We, as teachers and parents, are going to have to actively listen with the intent to understand, the ideas and perspectives of others. Parents bring a keen knowledge of their child, but, they are too often left on the sidelines - watching others plan for their child. Teachers bring years of experience teaching many children (sometimes thousands) as well as professional training in a variety of pedagogical approaches. We cannot discount their perspective.

If we want to implement a plan that will bring the student's Individual Education Plan to life every single day in the classroom, each one of us will need to use our skills as problem solvers, analyzers, organizers and team players! There is no place for personal agendas and ego. Educational planning for a child with Autism Spectrum Disorder must be authentic rather than generic; it must be ongoing rather than static; and it must reflect the individual's abilities and disabilities as well as the curriculum requirements. When we keep the plan individual, relevant and dynamic we are well on the way to making this school year a success!

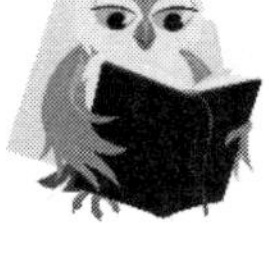

Every child deserves a champion – an adult who will never give up on them, who understands the power of connection and insists that they become the best that they can possibly be.

Rita Pierson

What Does Autism Spectrum Disorder Look Like in the Classroom?

Autism is a life-long, complex developmental disorder resulting from neurological differences in the functioning of the brain. These differences have a profound impact on the way a child thinks, behaves, communicates, learns and relates to the people in his or her life and the environment. Each and every child presents a unique expression of symptoms that often change over time. Sometimes, symptoms will manifest differently on a given day! As non–medical as it sounds, some individuals seem to have days where they seem 'more autistic' than on other days! Every parent of a child with autism knows that some days their children are more "off" and harder to figure out than other days. To be fair, it is often *our* lack of organization or planning that creates a 'more autistic day!"

To complicate matters further, individuals with autism often exhibit 'splinter skills:' a child may show above average intelligence in one area and below average in another domain. For example, a child might not respond when you ask his name but he will count to a hundred with little difficulty. Or a student may be able to compute complex mathematical equations and yet struggle immensely with making a prediction in a narrative story.

Autism is not always visibly noticeable, especially in those individuals that have advanced language skills and a more social nature. Metaphorically, autism is much like an iceberg: some children will exhibit odd behaviour, difficulty with speech and/or social interactions, but, these are just the 'tip of the iceberg.' Issues with thinking, verbal/ non-verbal communication, executive function, anxiety and sensory integration often hide beneath the 'surface' but have the potential to wreak havoc on the individual's overt functioning. Sometimes it isn't until we ask the student to choose a topic to write about, work in a group or play with peers that autism becomes more glaring.

It is inaccurate to judge the severity of an individual's autism based on what we see or fail to see. Sometimes the most 'typical' looking kid lives with some very challenging and invisible autism traits. At the same time, a student may appear to be very 'low functioning' and yet harbor hidden capabilities. Appearances can be brutally deceiving when it comes to autism. The range in severity, complexity and the changing nature of autism makes parenting and teaching these individuals both exhilarating and perplexing!

Our own son is one of those kids whose looks are deceiving: A bright, articulate boy with a brain that is significantly impacted by autism. When people meet him, many assume he has a very mild case of autism. (For the record, never, never, say <u>that</u> to parent of a child with special needs!) He is sociable, affectionate, and articulate. But, Kieran's walk to school may serve to illustrate the impact of autistic thinking on a kid who is very intelligent and does not 'look' autistic.

One morning my husband agreed to allow our son, aged 10, to walk to school rather than take the school bus. The school was a 15 minute walk straight north on the same street so my husband agreed to forego the usual 'practice sessions' (priming) that Kieran would typically do before he performed a skill independently. A few minutes after Kieran left home, my husband left in his car to secretly 'shadow' Kieran's walk. Much to his surprise, our boy was nowhere in sight! Stomach in his throat, Ivars began scouring the neighborhoods. Within a matter of minutes, Kieran was spotted - walking in a westward direction! Rolling down the car window and attempting to sound nonchalant, Ivars inquired as to where he was headed. Peering into the window with a perplexed look, Kieran gave a strikingly logical response: he was headed towards school, going exactly where the bus goes!

Ah, those are the moments when parents are once again reminded that autism has a sneaky way of influencing one's thought process! Our son's thinking was quite logical, but not very efficient. In fact, it may have added an hour or more to his 15 minute walk! Yes, even the most high- functioning, even-mannered individuals can be quite impacted in their thinking. Teachers need to be especially vigilant when assuming that a student is capable of higher level thinking and age appropriate behaviour because that may not be the case and - it certainly is not the child's fault!

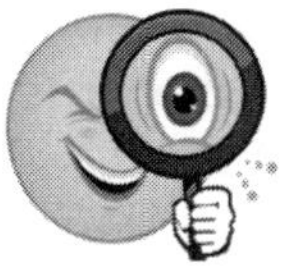

Autism: A Closer Look

Before we get into the 'nitty gritty' of what autism might look like in your classroom, I feel compelled to remind the reader that our kids with autism do not come to school to be cured. Autism is not a problem to be fixed. We are not called to be miracle workers or clinicians. Rather, our role is to identify and build on individual abilities and to teach skills that will facilitate autonomy, independence and self -esteem. Like all children, students with autism need their parents and teachers to teach them how to use their strengths in order to build bridges for their weaknesses and to grow to be more independent and autonomous. If we bring a deficit mentality of autism to our teaching we will certainly be overwhelmed in no time. If we are looking for a clear cut, 'one size fits all' educational solution for teaching a student with autism we might as well save our energy. Efforts we put into learning as much as possible about each individual child with autism and planning for that child based on his own interests, needs, and strengths will deliver more benefit for both teacher and student. Please don't ever forget that students with autism **will** progress when programs, resources and goals are matched to their unique needs and strengths.

Our kids with autism do not come to school to be cured. Autism is not a problem to be fixed.

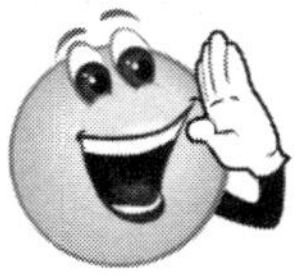

Students with autism WILL progress when programs, resources and goals are matched to their unique needs and strengths.

The Diagnostic Definition of Autism

In spite of the complex nature of Autism, the Diagnostic Statistical Manual – V outlines two areas of impairment for the diagnosis of Autism Spectrum Disorder.

A. Persistent deficits in social communication and social interaction across multiple contexts, as manifested by the following, currently or by history

- Deficits in social-emotional reciprocity
- Deficits in nonverbal communicative behaviours used for social interaction
- Deficits in developing, maintaining, and understanding relationships

Specify current level of severity

B. Restricted, repetitive patterns of behaviour, interests, or activities, as manifested by at least two of the following, currently or by history

- Stereotyped or repetitive motor movements, use of objects, or speech
- Insistence on sameness, inflexible adherence to routines, or ritualized patterns or verbal nonverbal behaviour
- Highly restricted, fixated interests that are abnormal in intensity or focus
- Hyper- or hyperactivity to sensory input or unusual interests in sensory aspects of the environment

Specify current level of severity

C. Symptoms must be present in the early developmental period (but may not become fully manifest until social demands exceed limited capacities, or may be masked by learned strategies in later life).

D. Symptoms cause clinically significant impairment in social, occupational, or other important areas of current functioning.

E. These disturbances are not better explained by intellectual disability (intellectual developmental disorder) or global developmental delay. Intellectual disability and autism spectrum disorder frequently co-occur; to make comorbid diagnoses of autism spectrum disorder and intellectual disability, social communication should be below that expected for general developmental level.

Severity Level:

Level 3
"Requiring very substantial support"
Level 2
"Requiring substantial support"
Level 1
"Requiring support"

DSM – V Diagnostic Criteria, Autism Speaks, retrieved on January 15, 2014 from http://www.autismspeaks.org/what-autism/diagnosis/dsm-5-diagnostic-criteria)

In its previous version, the Diagnostic Statistical Manual (DSM IV) outlined a triad of impairments for an Autism diagnosis: 1) Impairments in communication, 2) Impairments in social interactions and 3) Patterns of behaviour, interests and/or activities that are restricted, repetitive, or stereotypic.

The newest version - DSM V - describes the Autism diagnosis in two main areas: 1) deficits in social communication and social interaction and 2) restricted repetitive behaviours, interests, and activities. Under the DSM-V criteria, individuals with autism must show symptoms from early childhood, even if those symptoms are not recognized as ASD until later. Early identification is paramount and the latest version of the manual will hopefully help in that area. It will also acknowledge those individuals who meet the criteria for ASD at a later age.

Language and communication are so entrenched in social interactions that it seems reasonable to combine them into a single criteria.The decision to leave out a language delay, which was once a key feature of Autism, was largely due to the fact that these delays are not observed in all individuals with autism. Secondly, language delays can also be a symptom of so many different disorders.

Diagnostic Criteria

Impairments in Social Communication

Students on the autism spectrum have difficulty with both expressive and receptive communication. Receptive language ability should never be assumed for our students. They may, in fact, understand more (or less) of what we communicate. A student with autism may seem to understand a communicative message, but, the proof is shown if their response or actions match what they 'understand.' Repeating back a message is not the equivalent of understanding. When a student repeats your instruction to get the text from the library and come back to class but subsequently sits at his desk, he has failed to understand the message.

Given that our students with autism will likely be able to process simple information quite well and that they can 'talk a good game' we can sometimes be fooled by what we think they understand. At the risk of repeating myself: parents and educators must be cautious. We tend to overestimate the amount of language the student understands. We also use reasoning to explain a point. The problem is that people with autism are far more impaired in language and higher level thinking, like reasoning, that we may realize.

In the Cognition section of this book we will examine receptive understanding in greater detail but for now, it is important that educators are aware that our autistic students (including all levels of intelligence) will need more time to process what we say. They will need simple, direct instructions and visual support (words and/or pictures) to supplement what is verbal. Complex language, long winded explanations and negative directives such as, "Don't write in red pen," will only confuse and slow down information processing.

About 25% of individuals with autism are non –verbal. A few decades ago it was thought that about 50% of children with autism would remain non-verbal. What is critical for parents and teachers to understand is that non- verbal does not equal intellectual disability (NIH, 2010). The success stories of three non-verbal individuals testify to the value of never giving up on finding a voice for our kids with autism.

At the age of two, Carly Fleischmann was diagnosed with severe autism and an oral motor condition that prevented her from speaking. She was never expected to develop intellectually beyond the ability level of a small child. Years of intensive behavioural and communication therapy yielded modest results and it would have been easy to assume that Carly had reached a ceiling in her communication ability. However, at the age of ten, she had a breakthrough. "While working with her devoted therapists Howie and Barb, Carly reached over to their laptop and typed in "HELP TEETH HURT," much to everyone's astonishment. This was the beginning of Carly's journey toward self-realization (carlys voice.com)." Carly lives in Toronto, goes to a mainstream high school, takes gifted classes and passionately advocates for those living with autism. She is the author of *Carly's Voice.*

Born with autism, Jenna Lumbard never developed speech nor could she always understand what was said. However, she became a voracious reader and in grade two, armed with a keyboard and the help of a facilitator, Jenna began to express ideas in poetry and short stories. Like Carly, Jenna wants to use her voice to inspire others to persevere and be the best they can be. Jenna has published, *Worried Wendy Goes to School.*

Our most critical task as parents and educators is to find a way to give a voice to those persons who cannot speak

Diagnosed as "severe" or "low-functioning" autism, Tito Rajarshi Mukhopadhyay had almost no language skills when he was eleven years old. His vocalizations were approximations of words and he was completely dependent on his mother. She taught him to read and write by using an alphabet board. From the age of six years he had learned to write by himself using a pencil. From this humble beginning, Tito has a remarkable ability to use long words in complex sentences and to express philosophical thoughts about life in spite of being severely disabled. In fact, at twenty-five years old, Tito is the author of three books: *The Mind Tree*, *The Gold of the Sunbeams*, and *How Can I Talk If My Lips Don't Move?*

We can never give up in our quest to give a student a voice.

Imagine a particularly killer day at school. Your ability to keep teaching is dependent on the consumption of coffee. For some reason, you have no voice and no way to write- no way to tell your need for coffee. (I know some readers will be able to relate). A colleague senses something is wrong and kindly brings you a salad. Very nice – but not what you want. A sweet student brings you a glass of water and again, you are grateful but you really *need* a coffee. The principal arrives at the door with a pile of report cards that need editing. Exhausted, tense and frustrated, your mood gets edgy. The people around you write off your mood as being "grouchy" – maybe even, "inappropriate." But, you really aren't in a foul mood, you just need coffee!

Too often we get so caught up in trying to develop great educational and behaviour plans for kids with autism that we overlook the more basic human need – to be able to express our needs and thoughts. The anecdote above is silly in comparison to how unbelievably frustrating it must be for a person who is non-verbal to deal with verbal folks who don't get it! Carly, Jenna and Tito are just three individuals with autism that have snapped me out of my oblivion in regards to planning for expressive needs. These beautiful, intelligent and incredibly patient individuals have made it abundantly clear that our most critical task as parents and educators is to find a way to give a voice to those persons who cannot speak. The need to express our needs, desires and thoughts is the foundation of who we are as humans. It doesn't matter if you have tried augmentative communication, sign language or Picture Exchange System and it didn't work. DO WHATEVER IT TAKES. Keep working with others, keep asking questions and do not stop until you find a method (or more than one) that allows a student with autism to express who they are.

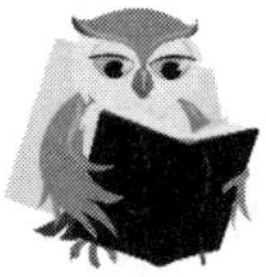

> ***"One of the most important pieces of ammunition people have for their own self - protection is the ability to ask and the ability to explain."***
>
> ***Donna Williams***

Within the autism diagnosis, there are individuals who will 'talk your ear off' and *appear* to be highly verbal. Educators beware! Being able to speak and sound articulate does not necessarily mean that what is being said reflects what the individual is trying to express. Too often we can mistake a student who talks a lot as a student who has strong oral communication skills. This is not always the case for students with autism. We must listen carefully to gain a sense of weaknesses in planning, vocabulary choice and even the ability to keep up with the speed of discourse in a conversation.

Understanding the ideas of others, what is read, and understanding the verbal and non - verbal actions of others can be frustrating. During a self-awareness interview conducted with a 16 year old boy with autism (who happens to be a seemingly strong oral communicator), the student expressed a high level of frustration in not being able to keep up with the pace of conversation amongst his peers. He explained that by the time he figured out what the teens were saying his retorts were ill timed. The teen admitted to being chastised for being slow on responding. He felt stupid (in spite of the fact that he is actually very bright).

The social deficits and difficulties that a student with autism experience are probably the most detrimental to self -esteem and the ability to be a fully participating member of a social group. These students invariably misunderstand or fail to acknowledge (in a timely manner) others' words, gestures and facial expressions. At times, they may even lack the motivation to engage in social interactions given the highly exhausting and unrewarding nature of social interaction. Socializing is a lot of work on the brain, especially when the social brain isn't hardwired efficiently.

Watching a child walk the perimeter of a school yard by himself has got to be one of the most heart wrenching sights for a parent and teacher. Older students may find ways to avoid the cafeteria and other social situations. One student described the situation to me as being akin to being a 'foreigner' in a strange land where the social nuances and language is unknown and the residents too impatient! If you have ever visited a foreign country or joined a social event in which you have little to no understanding of the language being spoken, you probably will be able to empathize! Imagine being expected to participate in meeting of neuroscientists. Personally, I would feel like a fish on a beach!

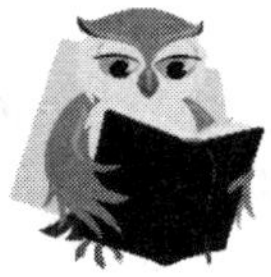

> ***The most basic of all human needs is the need to understand and be understood.***
>
> ***Ralph Nichols***

While some children with autism might seem 'anti- social,' others might be overly social. Failure to discriminate between friend and stranger in social initiatives can leave the individual with autism bewildered, or worse, vulnerable. Lack of discrimination can also be embarrassing. On one occasion, we were visiting a local car dealership and as the salesman approached us, our young son, bolted towards him, buried his head into the man's waist and bear hugged him! Stunned, the salesman nervously tousled the top of Kieran's head, coughed and chuckled. For Ivars and me, it was one of those moments in life when we say a silent prayer that a large hole in the floor will swallow us!

The following list describes some of the *possible* <u>social communication challenges</u> faced by students with autism:

- Delay in or lack of development of spoken language
- May use a lot of words but lacks understanding of what he/she is saying
- Difficulty initiating/sustaining conversation with others
- Failure to imitate the language and actions of others
- Difficulty regulating the volume of the voice
- Use of echolalic language (repeating words and phrases that may not have a functional use)
- Failure to use gestures (nodding head, pointing, shaking head) to express ideas
- Failure to respond when being spoken to or when name is called (hearing is normal)
- Idiosyncratic use of language or words (uses an expression or phrase when it doesn't make sense to do so)
- Failure to follow instructions (even after repeating the instructions verbatim)

- Difficulty answering questions or retelling narrative events in a coherent manner (what happened at recess)
- Difficulty understanding meaning in verbal instructions and reading
- Difficulty changing a subject in conversation if it is a topic of personal interest
- Misunderstanding figurative language (misunderstands jokes, idioms, metaphors and sarcasm - How can someone be as a mad as a hornet?)
- Misunderstanding of or inattention to others' non-verbal behaviours such as eye contact, facial expression, body postures and gestures to regulate social interaction (personal space, eye gaze)
- Failure to develop developmentally appropriate peer relationships (plays with children younger than self or gravitates to adults)
- May not seem very interested in sharing great news about school, home or a personal achievement
- May lack social or emotional reciprocity (may respond indifferently or oddly when others are crying, laughing, scared and so on)
- Lack of joint attention (following the gaze of or looking at where someone is pointing and failing to share a moment of sadness, excitement, joy or grief)
- Absence of eye contact and/or fleeting eye contact
- Does not initiate conversations or play with other students (may not know how to do so or may not be interested in doing so)
- Lack of meaningful friendships (particularly heartbreaking for parents)
- Uses inappropriate ways to gain the attention of other kids or adults (grabs or touches another person in inappropriate places, pulls hair, pushes a peer or just starts talking without gaining the other's attention first)
- Shows more interest in objects than in people
- Difficulty shifting attention between people, activities, visuals in the environment (this makes transition times or changes in routine excruciating at times)
- May lack understanding of others' emotions, thoughts, opinions and/or what causes them
- Difficulty in being an effective part of a group and working in a group
- Challenges in self- awareness and self- monitoring social behaviour and communication
- Difficulty keeping up with and processing the speed and complexity of a social conversation

More than any other autism characteristic, social communication challenges are the most detrimental to relationships and self- esteem. Non- autistic individuals can be impatient with social communication 'mistakes' because the processes that govern our social interactions are as innate and automatic as breathing itself – unless one has autism. It is easy to assume that an individual *should* know better! But, our students with autism cannot. It is also easy to underestimate the enormous energy drain that social interactions generate for individuals with autism. Social thinking is far more of an intellectual and conscious process for those who live with autism. It is no wonder that many might feel more comfortable staying out of the social arena!

What is perhaps most perplexing is that administrators and educators too often view social communication training as falling outside of the curriculum. It is absurd. Social challenges are the "elephant in the room" and sadly, if we don't acknowledge the necessity to work with kids in the messy and hard to teach realm of social thinking and relationships we will be missing the whole point! Behaviour problems, lack of academic development, anxiety and social isolation are the result. Unless we expect our students to live on an island alone, we cannot possibly prepare students for life after high school if we fail to address social communication education for students with autism.

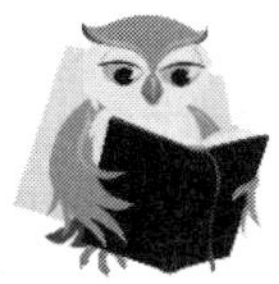

"The most important single ingredient in the formula of success is knowing how to get along with people."

Theodore Roosevelt

<u>Problems with Play</u>

Educators know that play time is essential for the development of all children. It helps them to develop language, social skills, thinking skills and leisure activities. Play gives children a chance to cultivate cognitive skills, flexible thinking, communication and creativity. It is far from a frivolous use of time. In essence, play is children's <u>work</u>!

Sadly, the ability to play is impaired in children with ASD. They don't seem to be wired to play 'properly' with toys or other children. Children with autism lack the prerequisite skills needed to use toys appropriately, to interact socially with a playmate and to use imagination in playing games. Pretend play seems to elude kids with ASD. Too often, repetitive behaviours get in the way of using a toy appropriately. A child may spin the tires of a toy car rather than 'drive' a toy car. For a child with autism, play can be eerily quiet. When typical kids crash two play cars, the result is often a loud vocalized, BAM! A student with autism does not seem to have a soundtrack attached to actions like crashing cars.

Autistic play often reveals a restricted or limited range of interests and play materials. Some kids with ASD show an attachment to unusual objects such as a spatula or a fishing lure - not exactly a toy that will attract a friend! For a child with ASD, strict adherence to rules may create friction and conflict with peers. Maybe little Beth insists on playing games by **her** rules or she breaks down when a playmate decides to play hopscotch rather than soccer. Little Bobby is only interested in sifting sand through his hands.

What might you see in your classroom?

- Lack of varied and spontaneous make-believe or social imitative play at the appropriate developmental level
- Failure to imitate what a peer or adult is doing with toys, body movements, or sounds
- Simple, repetitive nature of 'play': I.e. lining up, spinning or stacking objects; opening and closing doors
- Lack of play activities, unusual response to play objects (opens and closes a toy car door rather than 'driving it')
- Lack of parallel play and interactive play (does not interact with a child playing near him or with him)
- Lack of symbolic play (unable to pretend that a banana is a telephone or a stick is a sword
- Reliance on sensory manipulation of objects I.e. repeatedly feeling or smelling textures of toys
- Need for perfectionism
- Insistence that the environment or routine remain unchanged (won't allow you to move the toy cow from the barn)
- Lack of safety awareness with play materials (climbs too high, throws large objects)
- Tends to engage in solitary play or parallel play
- Failure to understand 'cause and effect' (if I hit the button, the bell rings)

Children with ASD need to learn *how* to play; it is a skill that is too important to ignore. In fact, play is the <u>foundation for all learning;</u> it is critical for a child's language, cognitive, emotional and social development.

In teaching play skills, the goal is to assist the child to expand his interests, use of language, imagination and to develop joint attention and symbolic play with toys. In a child's early years, we need to dedicate ourselves to developing play skills. We also want to help kids with autism to become desirable playmates for other children and to enjoy the world of play for themselves. We can increase the motivation to learn how to play by incorporating a child's strong interests into a more appropriate and adaptable play style. For example, a child who is fascinated by trains can be taught how to play with trains in an imaginative way so his peers may choose to share the interest in trains and play along. Playing boards games with train theme is another way to capitalize on an area of interest in order to expand skills.

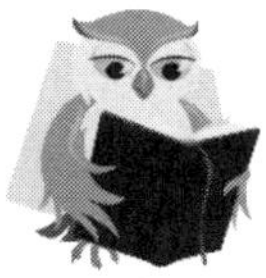

> ***"It is paradoxical that many educators and parents still differentiate between a time for learning and a time for play without seeing the vital connection between them."***
>
> ***Leo F. Buscaglia***

Patterns of Behaviour, Interests and/or Activities that are Restricted, Repetitive, or Stereotypic

If you have spent time with individuals with autism, you will have surely noticed that many have an extraordinary need for sameness. Let's be clear - this is a neurological hardwiring issue, not a personal choice. The need for sameness can be evident in an individual's need to preserve the daily schedule, the route taken to the gymnasium, and the placement and organization of objects within the classroom.

Furniture that has been rearranged, bulletin boards that have been updated or toys that are not in their proper place can throw an individual with autism into panic mode without warning! Our son always chose the same table in a restaurant, the same pew in church and the same spot at the kitchen table. I can remember my heart skipping a beat when we would notice someone eating at 'our table' at the local pizza place! It was a good thing Kieran was cute because he would march right over to the table and glare at the unsuspecting patrons! In response, they would often smile and try to divert this little man with small talk until we were able to orchestrate the rescue. At church Kieran was a little more vocal when he thought that someone had invaded our seat! "That's OUR seat!" he screeched on more than one occasion! Once he learned how to talk he made good use of the skill. Our children do have a knack of capitalizing on our self – consciousness as parents!

Rigid thinking is only one aspect of this group of diagnostic criteria. Repetitive body movements such as rocking, finger flicking, flicking lights, smelling objects or people and even more subtle movements are part and parcel of an autistic neurology. In the same way, an intense passion for particular and sometimes odd interests (as perceived from a neuro-typical perspective) can be indicative of a brain that is wired differently.

The following is a list of some of the behavioural patterns we <u>may</u> see in students with autism:

- Preoccupation with an area of interest that is abnormal either in intensity or focus (not abnormal because *we think* it is a weird interest)
- Inflexible need to stick to non-functional routines/rituals (must take the same route to the gymnasium or grocery store, or sit in the same seat in the library, or keep

the pencil case on the top, left of the desk) - may seem to a teacher that student is oppositional or defiant - Frustration and emotional upset results when routines and rituals are disrupted I.e. What do you mean the movie is sold out? The library HAS to be open!

- Insistence on sameness; demands that the bulletin board with his name remain there all year! Don't even think of rearranging that furniture or those desks!
- Repetitive motor or vocal mannerisms (e.g., hand wringing, finger flicking, rocking, smacking lips together repetitively, clicking sounds)
- Repetitive or unusual manipulation of objects and toys (turning the wheels of a toy car incessantly or repeatedly opening and closing a door on a toy barn)
- May get mentally stuck (constant repeating of a question or a response, inability to brainstorm a variety of options or solutions)
- May feel agitated or upset by seemingly minute changes in the environment or people (teacher's hair is NOT in a ponytail!)
- Self- injury (head banging, slapping self, biting)
- Strict adherence to rules - may become very agitated if weight restrictions are ignored in elevators, or if rules are changed in a game with peers or in physical education class and/or recess

Patterns of behaviour, interests and/or activities that are restricted, repetitive, or stereotypic are in large part due to neurological wiring that is far beyond the control of a person who lives with an autistic brain. It is beyond the scope of this book to accurately describe the theories of why the autistic brain manifests the symptoms of autism. And yet, it is critical that those involved with autistic individuals understand that in the mind of a person with autism, rules give structure and predictability in a world where there seems to be none. Rules are a cornerstone of safety. If everything around me feels out of control and if my perceptions only make my world fragmented, then I live in a state of constant anxiety; my routines, rituals, and rules make me feel safe and secure.

Given the brain differences in autism, neuro- typical people cannot pretend to comprehend the degree of confusion and intensity of the internal world the same way an autistic person experiences it. But, I think it helps to reflect on situations where we may feel a loss of control in order to build understanding and empathy. Think about someone you know who needs to have an itinerary or hotels booked before she can enjoy a trip. How many of us need to know ahead of time when our workshop will schedule a break and lunch. We may even be anxious to know what will be served for lunch so that we can plan to an alternative. Imagine playing a sport where they were no rules and no referees maintaining some semblance of order and safety. Consider those times when the traffic lights at a major intersection are not working and disarray follows. Many parents will start to 'lose it' if laundry is on the sofa, dishes are in the sink, and coats on the floor. The need for some sense of organization and control is in all of us to varying degrees. We are most vulnerable and least adept of self -control when life situations are out of our control.

A non- autistic mind might view the autistic's need to follow rules as a behaviour problem. True, rules can be a little *too* restrictive at times. Children playing at recess tend to get aggravated by an overzealous rule cop. So too, are teachers who experience the unwillingness of a student to ride on a bus with no seat belts - even if it is for a field trip. On a hot summer day when we were looking forward to spending a day boating with friends, our 11 year old son insisted that we could not possibly go out in the boat because we were going to exceed the weight restriction (which we were not). No amount of explanation from his police officer (marine unit) father would help Kieran to understand that some rules are guidelines and we were well within the safety guidelines for our boat. We did not *need* to weigh our guests before they got in the boat! Tears, frustration and worn patience almost ruined a fun outing. The necessity of following rules was less than amusing this time!

What does the term behaviour mean to you?

Does the mere mention of the word behaviour automatically conjure a mental image of a child acting disruptively or inappropriately? If so, you are not alone. To some degree, I think that we all hold negative connotations associated with the term 'behaviour'.

But, the fact is, that 'behaviour' is not necessarily negative or positive; it just is what it is. Behaviour is anything a person says or does; buying a coffee, sending an email, waving goodbye are all 'behaviours.' So too, are swearing, kicking, biting and screaming. The difference comes down to the fact that some behaviours are more obnoxious, disruptive and annoying than others. Some we would like to increase and others, decrease.

Everything we do or say serves a purpose. The purpose comes from our thinking. If I want to decrease a behaviour (or increase it), I need to know what purpose it is serving. Why do I incessantly check my iphone? Why am I always late for work on Monday mornings? Why do I bite my nails? Why do I have to have coffee first thing in the morning? Our actions are driven by a purpose. Our purpose is driven by the thoughts that we hold and the neurological wiring of our brains.

I admit that I for one get really tired of hearing the adage, "behaviour is communication." This is especially true in the midst of an exhausting day with a student who is unravelling before my eyes! During those episodes at the pizza place and at church, I certainly was not inclined to interpret what our son was telling us! In the heat of the moment, shrouded in embarrassment, I was too busy trying to put out the fire to honestly care why he was acting the way he was! Eventually, when the calm returns and the heartbeat regulates, we are usually more willing to look for the message behind the behaviour. More than ever before, we know that the message is derived from autistic thinking.

The more we understood his autistic mind, the better we understood that our son's 'rudeness' arose from his neurologically hardwired need for sameness. His little world felt like it would collapse when it was abruptly changed. As adults we can convince ourselves that when a child acts up, it is a sign that the child needs to change. Truth be told, tantrums, meltdowns and unexpected behaviours are our cue that we need to do some homework. Parents and educators will be much more effective when we seek to understand what thoughts are driving the behaviour so that we can respond to the message and teach an alternative way to send the message.

For example, if in my mind, I feel as though I am overwhelmed by a messy and disorganized house I tend to become more controlling - a 'micro manager' - my husband would say. Experience has taught him that no amount of telling me to relax and take a break will ease my behaviour and make me easier to live with. My thinking affects my behaviour. If my family wants to reduce the beahviour it is wise to change what happens *before* the potential behaviour (antecedent) or *after* it occurs (consequences). Tidying and cleaning have a magical effect on my behaviour – especially when done BEFORE my anxiety rises! It is less effective when completed AFTER my behaviour. This personal example hopefully illustrates that we all exhibit less than endearing 'behaviour' at times. This is not solely an autistic characteristic! However, for individuals with autism (as we shall see in the section on cognition) autistic thinking is complex and if we want to modify behaviour it is essential that we become familiar with the ways autism impacts thinking.

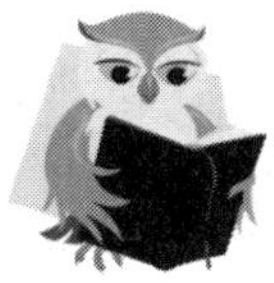

"When something is 'all in your mind' people tend to think that it is willful, that it's something you could control if you tried harder or you had been trained differently. I am hoping that the newfound certainty that autism is in your brain and in your genes will affect public attitudes."

(Grandin, 2013, p. 204)

Once we have a better understanding of the thinking producing behaviour, we are able to teach skills and use strategies to instill more appropriate ways to express a need. Expecting behaviour to change because, 'we say so,' is futile. Over time we came to understand that inflexible thinking (due to wiring problems in the brain) was most likely the source of Kieran's stress when someone was sitting in 'his' seat. With visual teaching using Social Stories™, social scripts and picture rehearsal Kieran was able to tolerate someone else in 'his' seat. This behaviour served as a signal that he needed help with developing flexible thinking.

As adults in the world of the child with autism, we have a threefold task:

1. Determine what the behaviour is telling us about the student's cognitions and thinking.

2. Identify what we need to do to respond to the message. We have three options (usually we address all three).

   First, address the **person**. What skills need to be taught? For example, how we can facilitate a more acceptable way for the child to communicate his needs?

Second, address the **task**. Is the task asking the student to work in an area of deficit? What supports are needed to scaffold the task completion? Is it too demanding/too easy? Are there prerequisite skills that need to be taught?

Third, address the **environment**. Is there a plan and space for "calming?" Does the organization of materials and space facilitate independent movement and access to resources? Are materials available for students to address individual sensory needs, not contingent on behaviour or performance?

3. Fade out adult assistance (work ourselves out of a job). Facilitate generalization of skills with different people, a variety of materials or content and in different situations.

Human behaviour is driven by our needs. The main messages that we can read from behaviour are:

I need your attention. (Negative or positive will do!)

I need something tangible. (Toys, food, activities, structure, a plan, etc…)

I need to escape or avoid something. I need to change something. (The task, the environment, the "scratchy" shirt, the activity, the transition, the person sitting too close to me, the challenging work, the shame of feeling incompetent, having to wait, disappointment, etc…)

I need to self -regulate. (Sensory needs: I need to feel my body in space, and/or find my balance, and/or touch, smell, taste, sight or touch something)

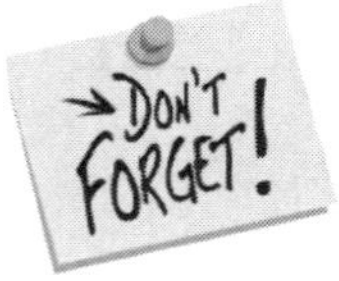

Don't forget to consider:

Sensory/Non-social (Automatic) – Are there situations in which behaviour is maintained independent of the social environment such as in a room, alone?

Medical/Physical – Is an underlying medical condition or physical pain causing distress?

In the personal example of my over controlling, micro managing behaviour I would argue that all of the above messages were at play:

My thoughts told me (erroneously) that I needed to nag more and control more in order to get my family's attention and express my own needs for order and cleanliness (attention). My behaviour was my attempt to get them to tidy and clean (tangible). A brain injury causes a neurology that demands order and structure in order to reduce anxiety. I would even say that I was trying to escape the burden of feeling overwhelmed and frenzied.

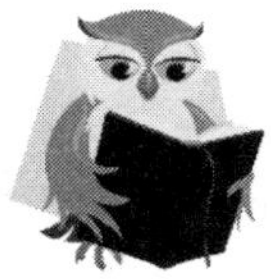

> **"If you just learn a single trick, Scout, you'll get along a lot better with all kinds of folks. You never really understand a person until you consider things from his point of view... until you climb inside of his skin and walk around in it."**
>
> **Atticus Finch in *To Kill a Mockingbird*, Harper Lee**

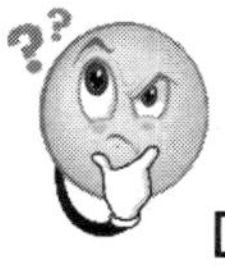

My Student Doesn't Have any Behaviour Problems!

Don't be fooled! A student who is sitting quietly, displaying absolutely no 'behaviour' may need our attention just as much, or more than the student who is screaming and banging his head! Sitting quietly may indicate that the child is off in another world, completely oblivious to the lessons being taught. This child needs us to teach self –monitoring and to increase his motivation to stay on task. Unfortunately, the louder and more destructive a student is, the more attention they receive! Similarly, a student who wanders the perimeter of a school yard at recess may be well behaved, but, her behaviour indicates to staff that she needs support friendship and probably skill training. Behaviour does not have to be deemed "inappropriate" in order to call for intervention.

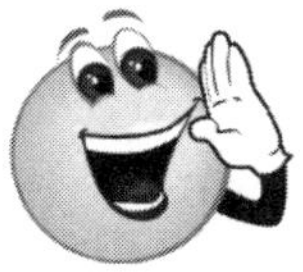

> ***Behaviour does not have to be deemed "inappropriate" in order to call for intervention.***

<u>*Unusual Responses to Sensory Experiences*</u>

The impact sensory dysfunction has on our children with autism cannot be overstated. It is difficult for those with a non - autistic brain to fathom what sensory dysfunction does to unravel individuals. Social interactions, eating, sleeping, behaviour and a sense of well -being can be drastically affected by sensory dysfunction. To get a tiny inkling of what this might feel like, consider what it is like to try to fall asleep or concentrate when the room is extremely hot or cold. Are you able to carry on a conversation in a crowded pub with a punk band screaming from the stage? Have you ever tried to focus on finishing a project when you had vertigo? When the waistline of your pants is cutting into your skin, do you find yourself agitated? Have you attempted to listen attentively to a friend on the phone while her toddler screams in the background? Are you able to thoroughly appreciate nature while walking in the woods with hordes of mosquitoes hovering around you? What's wrong? Just relax. Just ignore the distractions. Try harder.

Not exactly helpful responses are they?

Individuals who do not experience sensory challenges as individuals with autism do, can be somewhat arrogant and unaccommodating in our responses. Sometimes we expect autistic kids to ignore stimuli or focus harder without helping them to cope with their sensory issues. Don't forget that while we may be able to name what is aggravating us or interrupting our attention, many individuals with autism cannot identify or articulate the culprit. Even if they are able to recognize the problem, too often, they lack the adaptive, language and/or executive function skills to fix the issue.

Students with autism may be trying to cope with all sorts of sensory difficulties while being expected to think, communicate and behave appropriately. People living with constant pain, ringing in their ears, brain injury, vertigo or chronic headaches may have a sense of what I am trying to make clear. Everything in their experience is affected by these difficulties.

Sensory difficulties usually come in two categories. The first, is a HYPER (too much) sensitive response to stimulation. The second, is a HYPO (too little) response to sensory stimulation. In a hypo - sensory state, the student's body would be overwhelmed by a constant invasion of sensory impulses. The brain has no filters and senses too much. On the other hand, that same child may not receive enough information from another sense (hypo sensory), leaving him or her in dire need of stimulation in order to feel anything. Sensory difficulties may help to explain odd reactions and behaviour. Sensory sensitivities can cause the child to act hyper-vigilantly or under responsively. The student may be anxious and easily distracted by lights, sounds and smells that most of us cannot even perceive. Signs of sensory difficulties can include aggression, head banging, self-injury and screaming.

I have taught students who appeared to have no need for warm clothing in cold temperatures. It was always a struggle to convince them to wear a hat, coat and boots rather than a T shirt and flip flops in the dead of winter. Kieran would show little or no sign of pain as a child. He could be covered in blood with a nasty gash and he would seem unaware that there was a problem. Bailey, a teen girl, could not stand the slightest touch unless she initiated it. On the other hand, when she did initiate touch she would throw her body at you and wrap her arms so tightly around the upper body that it hurt. Derrick, another student, would scream, "That hurt!" if I brushed past him. Brad would wince and wave his hands wildly upon entering the school. In darker rooms his whole body relaxed. These are not ill behaved students. They are kids with autism that suffer from mixed - up sensory systems. Temple Grandin recalls:

"As far back as I can remember, I always hated to be hugged. I wanted to experience the good feeling of being hugged, but it was just too overwhelming. It was like a great engulfing tidal wave of stimulation and I reacted like a wild animal. Being touched triggered flight; it flipped my circuit breaker. I was overloaded and would have to escape, often by jerking away suddenly" (Grandin 1995 p. 62).

In 1991, Laura Cesaroni and Malcolm Garber, at the Ontario Institute for Studies in Education, interviewed a twenty - seven year old male, a male aged thirteen and his parents. The study aimed to explore the experience of autism through firsthand accounts. Both males, experienced multi - channeled sensory processing. The older participant described his difficulty with hearing and seeing at the same time. It is hard to imagine, but sound came through as colour for this man. At the same time, touching something produced a sound sensation.

The children that I have taught tended to be more mono channel. If asked to give eye contact, many demonstrated that their ability to hear declined. Or vice versa. This demonstrates that it is impossible to judge the way another person experiences the world. Your student may present much less intrusive sensory difficulties than some described in this book. No two people with autism are alike. However, it is critical that the sensory difficulties a child with autism experiences should never be discounted or underestimated.

One of the best ways to support students and grow professionally (and personally) is to read autobiographies of individuals living with autism and sensory challenges. A reading list is included in the Appendices.

A closer look at each sensory system:

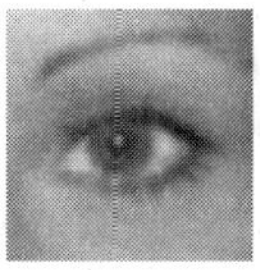

The Visual System

When a baby is still very new, he learns about his world through his sense of touch. The visual system is still very underdeveloped. A baby will wrap his little fingers around your finger if you touch his hand, but he will not yet, look at your finger. When the child finally looks at your finger after he grabs it, he is using his tactile system to direct his visual system. Eventually the baby will reach out and grab an object in his near vicinity. By the time a child is about six months of age, while holding an object; she will turn it around and examine it with her eyes. Her vision system is developing automatically.

Individuals with autism may have 20/20 eyesight but vision development is not as automatic as it is in typical persons. Some children with autism are still living with the visual system of a newborn. Their bodies are directed by their tactile system. But their world is limited to objects that they can see within one's grasp. If a child cannot touch it, he cannot see it. In these instances, the tactile system is still directing the body and the brain. The child may be in constant motion and not in control of where he is in space. Picture an infant, whose legs and arms are moving ceaselessly with no sense of direction. Eventually, that baby will gain a sense of control over his own body. For a child with autism, the visual experience can be very similar to that of a baby. The child may need a firm touch on the shoulder or a weighted vest (with OT approval) to gain a sense of where he is in relation to a chair.

Over years, a typical person's visual system matures and it takes on its usual role of directing the body and the brain. As language develops, the child learns to name specific objects he is able to see. He can visualize an object without physically seeing it. Words like, truck, table, bed and pizza each have an image associated with them, even when they are not present. By the age of ten, the goal of a sensory system is always integration. By taking information from all points of entry (eyes, ears, skin, mouth and so on) and synthesizing that input, it directs the body to respond appropriately. One way to understand integration is to think of accomplishing the ultimate sensory integration challenge - being able to place your body into a canoe without landing in the water!

As the visual system matures, we begin to understand things about objects without actually touching them. For example, most of us know that ice cream is cold without having to touch it. The development of vision is integrated with the development of language, motor and cognitive skills. With fully developed eyesight we gain the ability to distinguish the relationship between size and distance. Vision, goes beyond the way our eyes function. It is the ability to understand what we see, store the information, and retrieve what we have seen at a later time.

Autism can have a dramatic effect on the development of the visual system. Not all individuals with autism have immature visual systems, but, many have visual patterns that interfere with their ability to interact and respond to their environment. Temple Grandin explains that some autistic individuals experience "whiteouts" where vision completely shuts down. Depth perception problems can leave a person debilitated. (Grandin 1995, p. 73). Other visual problems may include (but are not limited to) avoidance of eye contact, poor and uneven handwriting, inability to listen and look simultaneously, overuse of peripheral vision, a stiff-legged walk, inability to catch a ball, and poking at the sides of the eyes. Visual abnormalities may draw a child to intensely bright lights or to flicking objects in front of his or her eyes.

Impaired vision affects such skills as eye-hand coordination, eye-foot coordination, eye movement control, convergence, difficulty with eye contact and eye-hand-foot-brain coordination. Vision skills impact a child's ability to eat without spilling, walk without falling, and to catch a ball without being hit by it. Poorly developed vision affects a child's penmanship, reading, attention span and socialization skills. It is really important to be aware of these possible vision challenges in order to understand that your student(s) may be "seeing" and experiencing the world differently than you are. Differences in visual patterning can cause the child to appear to be lazy, defiant or poorly behaved. As he matures, our son presents with higher functioning autism than when he was young. He is able to participate reasonably well in some sports, socialize with friends and function well in school. But, his visual perceptions impact some aspects of his life. For example, if asked him to vacuum a room or paint a wall he cannot cover a whole surface area. Left on his own, he will go over the same small area repetitively. Even after instruction and modeling, it is obvious that he has a hard time. In school, when asked to sketch a scene or a prototype, our 14 year old boy would inadvertently create his sketch or scene in a small corner of the paper. Visual perceptual assessments explained this behaviour – it wasn't merely a "guy thing" as some tried to point out.

Asking Kieran to search for something is often futile. Although he sweeps the room with his eyes, an object can be right in front of him and he will not see it. He really can't see it. Many people know non - autistic persons with the same problem. However, in individuals with autism, it is far more of a sensory processing issue than avoidance behaviour. We would not define a visually impaired person as lazy or defiant for not being able to see something that is right in front of their eyes. It would be unfair to judge a person with autism for their visual patterns.

In her book, *Thinking in Pictures: My Life with Autism,* Dr. Temple Grandin writes: "*If visual processing problems are suspected, the child should see a developmental optometrist. This is a special eye doctor who can do therapy and exercises to help the processing problems that are inside the brain. In many of these children, the eye itself is normal but faulty wiring in the brain is causing the problem"* (Grandin 2006, p. 79).

The following is a simple chart outlining some more of the more common characteristics of the visual system that persons with autism may experience.

Visual System	**HYPER Sensitive**	**HYPO Sensitive**
This is the system in our body that receives information through our sight.	Avoids or is sensitive to sunlight, bright lights (extreme aversion to light) Attends to (or may be distracted by) shiny objects or light effects Some are able to see the gas streaming through a fluorescent light! May look 'through' objects rather than 'at' objects May use peripheral vision (reads or examines an object from the periphery of his eyes) May sweep the room with eyes but not look at specific objects Looking through or beyond objects Lack of reciprocal play (throwing/catching a ball) Inordinate fear of heights or lack of appropriate fear of heights	Unaware of changes in lighting or the presence of other people Stares Turns objects right in front of the eyes Fascinated with moving objects and mirrors Rocking /jumping/swinging

The following information illustrates very effectively the kinds of visual patterns that may exist for some folks on the autism spectrum.

Peripheral vision is using side vision. You can get the feeling of peripheral vision by putting your hand in front of your face and looking around your hand. Some individuals with autism shift from the extreme right to the extreme left, moving the head as the eyes shift. This results in picking up fragments of visual information, instead of the full picture. Some individuals with autism switch from peripheral to central vision. Put your hand, once again, in front of your face. Separate your fingers in the center of your hand. Now switch from side to side or look at a detail in the center. The visual information is still fragmented.

Scanning or darting is that constant shifting or sweeping motion. Again, put your hand in front of your face and continue to shift your eyes from one position to another. You may notice objects in the room jump at you, swim, blur, or double. The act of constantly scanning can lead to dizziness, headaches, nausea and disorientation.

Seventy percent or more of individuals with autism do not automatically develop an efficient **binocular (**two-eyed) pattern. Think of the eyes as being two cameras. They need to point, focus, move exactly to avoid blur or double vision. When the two do not work exactly as a team, the individual experiences blur or double vision, or the brain conveniently suppresses vision partially or totally. Total suppression of an eye eliminates some visual confusion but does not allow information to get to both sides of the brain. Partial suppression leads to much confusion and visual stress making all visual tasks exhausting.

Poor visual attention: When the visual system is working correctly, the individual can see, understand what is seen, and remember what is seen with speed, accuracy, at any time and with little energy. An inefficient system makes controlling the eyes difficult. Shifting with exactness, and maintaining clear eyesight becomes exhausting. The physical effort is extensive, leaving little energy to understand, remember or use what was seen. (Fields of Vision, 1996)

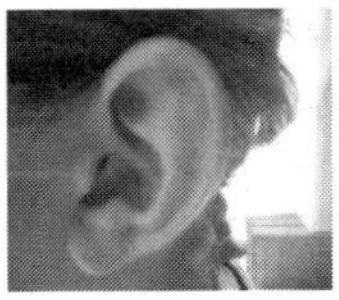

The Auditory System

Many students with autism will have normal hearing but they will experience trouble in processing information that comes in through their ears. In her book, *The Autistic Brain*, Temple Grandin speaks of her own auditory processing challenges in terms of a language input problem. As a child, Temple, had a difficult time differentiating between quick consonant sounds such as, 'p, c, and h' in the words pat, cat and hat. These sounds are spoken quickly and softly making them hard to differentiate. Grandin also struggled with a speech output problem in that when she was able to understand what people were saying to her sometimes the words got stuck as she tried to respond. Slowing down her speech was the only way to manage this difficulty (Grandin 2013, p.83).

In addition, Dr. Grandin describes other types of auditory processing problems common in persons with autism. Hearing words but being unable to connect any meaning to them is one example. I can relate to this when I am in another country, immersed in a language that I hear very well, but understand very little! I may cope well until I need to understand in order to get directions, find a doctor or supplies!

Another challenge arises when one needs to shift attention from a sound heard in the environment back to what was being said or done. Any teacher who has attempted to teach and hold children's attention during construction or maintenance in the school can probably relate to how effortful shifting attention can be at times. Those individuals with autism and auditory processing challenges in this area must find environmental sounds, or sensory aggravating sounds to be disastrous with their thinking.

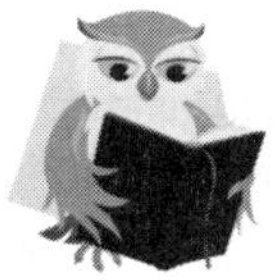

> ***"I found it difficult to concentrate when other children were talking among themselves…I find it hard to filter out external noise and regularly put my fingers in my ears to help me concentrate."***
>
> ***(Tammet, 2007, p. 80)***

Auditory processing problems can be very frustrating because it is easy to think that the child is ignoring us or failing to try hard enough. But this is not necessarily the case. Students with autism notoriously have poor auditory skills and higher visual skills. The key for us as educators and parents is to catch ourselves over relying on the child's auditory channels in communication. Are you explaining things verbally? Repeating yourself ad nauseam? Giving instructions verbally? Making small talk at the same time as you are expecting the individual to complete a task? Is there a lot of talking, whispering or noise in the individual's learning environment?

Individuals with autism may struggle to listen effectively if two people are talking at once. Too many voices in the background also impairs listening and attention. The brain gets confused and the listener is unable to pay attention to one voice. Noisy group work, classrooms and busy places may be too much to bear. Poor auditory processing may mean that the student hears only a few words rather than the whole sentence. Some persons with autism have described changes in volume while they listen. Imagine the frustration of having someone vary the volume of the radio while you are trying to hear important news.

Auditory System	**HYPER Sensitive**	**HYPO Sensitive**
This is the system in our body that receives information through our hearing.	Hears things that others cannot perceive (jets in the distance) Disturbed by "normal" sounds such as trains, mufflers, tunnels, children playing, seat belt reminders, fax machines, printers, vacuums, crowds, toilets) Creates repetitive sounds (may be an attempt to block out unpleasant sounds) Intensely troubled by fire alarms, alarm clocks (may respond physically if the sound is perceived as a threat) Easily distracted by background noises (a fan, pencils moving on paper, the scratch of chairs on the floor etc…)	Appears deaf (may not respond to name being called) Seeks repetitive or constant sounds, opening and closing doors, traffic, vacuum cleaners, fans, flushing the toilet, washing machines) Creates loud noises with objects or his own voice

The following are simple ways to compensate for auditory processing difficulties:

- ✓ Use visual organizers, labels, written copies of instructions, steps and schedules, concrete objects and every kind of visual method to supplement verbal information
- ✓ Provide plenty of processing time after you have spoken (once you repeat the question you are starting the whole processing time over!)
- ✓ Keep verbal instruction to a minimum: we mix up the input when we say too much
- ✓ Teach self- advocacy skills so that a child is able to express his or her need for processing time, visual supports and cues
- ✓ Minimize background sounds when the student is expected to think, talk or carry out a task

Auditory problems are very real for some individuals with autism. It is essential that we respect this fact and help the child in whatever way possible.

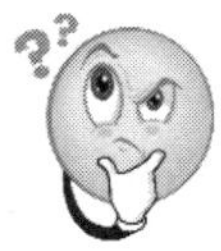

Are you explaining something verbally? Giving long instructions verbally? Making small talk at the same time as you are expecting the child to complete a task? Giving a directive and then explaining your reasons?

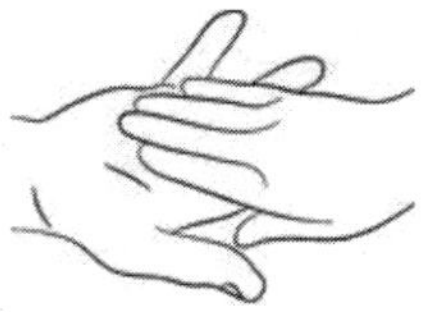

The Tactile System

Have you arrived at work only to realize that the clothes you chose were really irritating? Perhaps a bra strap that refuses to stay on your shoulder, a wool sweater making you itchy, or a tight waistband cutting off blood flow? As the day wore on you became increasingly aware of this feeling and it was driving you nuts! Maybe you wished you could race home and change or just remove the item of clothing that was annoying you!

Sometimes kids with autism feel the same way about their own *skin*! Unfortunately, skin is not removable. Some individuals with autism have reported feeling as if insects are biting them, bees are stinging them or something is digging into their skin. Not many of us would be able to go about our daily errands and business if that is how we felt. I for one, would be very irritable!

Many individuals with autism experience sensitivity to touch or tactile experiences. Several of the children I have taught have been highly sensitive to a sign of affection; recoiling from a hug or a gentle touch is quite common. Our son has never been comfortable standing in line where people are touching each other. Just as an amplifier magnifies sounds from musical instruments, autism can amplify normal and otherwise harmless tactile sensations. Behaviour problems can ignite over unknown or startling sensations. Stripping down to nakedness, screaming, bolting, and aggression are signs of overloaded tactile sensations.

Parent can be very proactive: removing tags from clothing, washing clothes or warming boot liners and mittens in the dryer before they are worn. I always ran my hand on the inside of an article of clothing before I purchased it for our son. To be sure he could wear it. Rough seams, zippers, or silk - screen would irritate him and lead to behaviour problems. When I found clothes that worked for him, I would buy several of the same items.

It is easy for adults to fall into the trap of believing that the child is seeking attention or just being silly or defiant because he rejects certain foods or flinches when a hand is placed on his shoulder. We can get frustrated when a student complains that another is touching him. I get it. Some kids DO want attention. Some are whiny! But, when a student has autism we simply cannot make those assumptions.

Tactile System	**HYPER Sensitive**	**HYPO Sensitive**
This is the system in our body that receives information through the skin, which picks up signals and tells us about touch, vibration, pressure, temperature and pain.	Avoids being touched, hugged Avoids certain textures in mouth or on hands (playdough, finger paint, glue) Avoids certain clothes (tags, textures, silk screen) Dislikes large groups of people and being bumped into (school hallways, malls at Christmas etc…) Removes clothing (now that's embarrassing!) Overreacts to insignificant injuries Hair brushing/cutting is often a nightmare Finger nail cutting is strongly disliked	Little or no sense of personal space High pain threshold Enjoys pressure….may be overly "huggy" Enjoys rough and tumble play (seeks it) Likes tight clothing or heavy blankets

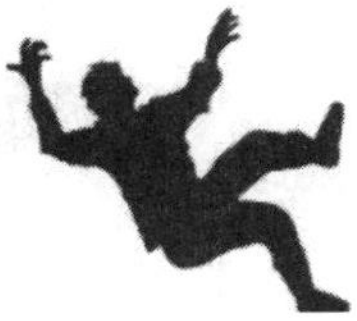

The Vestibular System

The vestibular system refers to structures within the inner ear that detect movement and changes in the head position. Even with your eyes closed, the vestibular system can tell you when your head is upright or tilted. It tells you whether you are stationary or moving, your direction and speed and whether objects around you are moving or still. Anyone who has ever struggled with balance and coordination knows how the vestibular system impacts these experiences. A mild brain injury gave me a taste of what life is like with an impaired vestibular system. It is not fun. We have a tendency to bump into things, trip and spill things, when we feel unsure of where our body is in space. We are called clumsy. Children with dysfunctional vestibular systems may exhibit odd behaviours or reactions to things that are believed to be harmless.

Vestibular System	**HYPER Sensitive**	**HYPO Sensitive**
This is the system in our body that receives information through movement and our sense of gravity.	Fearful of equipment or surfaces that move (may have trouble learning to climb or descend stairs or hills and they may be apprehensive walking or crawling on uneven or unstable surfaces) Avoids movement activities, active play (may appear lethargic) Moves close to walls, fences, railings and outer edges of areas Rigid body positions (may appear to have a tense pose or a fixed pose) Easily disoriented Fearful reactions to ordinary movement activities (e.g., swings, slides, ramps, inclines	They are trying continuously to stimulate their vestibular systems Seeks constant movement (may never seem to stay still!) Difficulty switching from a moving activity (especially to a stationary activity) Excessive body whirling, jumping, spinning, swirling, rocking

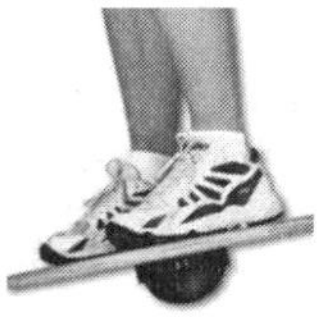

The Proprioceptive System

The proprioceptive system is responsible for the *unconscious* perception of movement or spatial orientation. The input or stimuli comes from within the body and it includes muscle and joint movements. Motor planning (also called praxis) develops when the tactile, vestibular and proprioceptive systems run properly in our bodies. When these three systems integrate, we are able to execute any physical task such as picking up a pencil, stepping into a canoe (and not falling into the water), catching a ball, riding a bike and so on. It is not uncommon to witness students with autism struggling to get these three systems to cooperate long enough to act on an idea or a need. Students can become “stuck” executing the simple task of moving from one spot in the classroom to another. It would be easy to assume the child is super stubborn. But, this situation is definitely not a matter of mind over matter. The brain’s failure to cooperate and communicate in different areas wreaks havoc on the body. Sometimes, it is helpful to write out the steps of what needs to happen. Feet on floor. Stand up. Walk to desk. Sit down. Open lunch bag. Small, manageable steps visually presented do the work that the brain should be doing!

When the proprioceptive system is working correctly, we *know* (unconsciously) where we are in space (our body position) and the position of our body parts in relation to other people and objects. Our body's position automatically adjusts in situations such as, sitting properly in a chair, stepping off a curb without tumbling over, writing with a pencil, using a fork to eat dinner and buttoning a sweater. It is difficult for most of us to write our name backwards. This is because we do not have a motor plan for this action. When I am learning an aerobics routine I look exceedingly spastic until my body gets accustomed to the sequence of movements and to where it is in space. For me, it is often necessary to teach a motor plan in small incremental steps and then repeat it numerous times so that my brain and the body finally have a solid pathway to follow when executing an action. Even then, my presentation is far from pretty! My dancer daughters obviously cannot attribute their grace to me!

What if many of the things you wanted to do felt the same way as writing your name backwards? Would you become frustrated? Would you be more likely to quit trying? Would <u>you</u> exhibit some inappropriate behaviours?

Difficulty with fine motor skills such as handwriting, colouring, and cutting with scissors are common challenges for some with autism. So too, is the need for perfection in the formation of letters or the struggle to feel the pencil in his or her hand or on the paper. Often, letters are poorly formed and larger than they should be. A child can become so frustrated at the amount of energy and concentration required to write a sentence or a word, that he has little hope of writing more than the minimum requirement. Even **that** may take an inordinate amount of time.

In the same manner we build large muscles with weight bearing exercise, we need to provide the child with fine motor activity practice. Incorporating a variety of fine motor activities into a young child's schedule will help to develop to strengthen these muscles, practice co-ordination and develop eye/hand co-ordination is definitely worth the time and effort. However, I become very concerned when parents or teachers put too much emphasis on the child's handwriting development. I have seen kids forced to stay in at recess, practice at home instead of playing outside, and I have seen children cry with the discomfort of printing and handwriting. Considering all of the areas of impairment that a child with autism faces, I think it is overkill to make the child practice at a skill that just makes them feel lousy about themselves. There are plenty of other skills that will have far reaching results in a child's life. Handwriting is not one of them.

In an age where computer literacy, touch screens and keyboarding are the norm we should spend time teaching a child how to use a keyboard and isolate the pointer finger to swipe a screen and tap an icon. While printing and handwriting are important too, developing these skills should not be overemphasized, especially when a child is able to produce more written output in less time on a keyboard.

Problems with catching and throwing a ball are common with some kids with autism. We know that the motor planning in these activities is quite complex. Children with autism may need one on one help to learn the basics. A skilled and compassionate buddy may be interested in coaching a student with autism (privately) making schoolyard and neighborhood games more enjoyable. To help teach these skills to our young son, my husband and I hired a male high school student to hang out with him, for a few hours a day in the summer months. Graham was far more patient and fun to be with than we were!

Please keep in mind that vision problems may negatively impact ball, sports and play skills.

Proprioceptive System	**HYPER Sensitive**	**HYPO Sensitive**
This system gives us a sense of where a certain body part is and how it is moving.	Clumsy movements Trouble with coordination Avoids crunchy or chewy foods Seems to be weak or not athletic Avoids hugs, touch or deep pressure Difficulty in handwriting – illegible printing	Clumsy movements Prefers tight clothing, heavy blankets (weighted blankets and vests) May prefer hard, crunchy foods May bite non-edibles Seeks deep pressure, squeezes or hugs hard

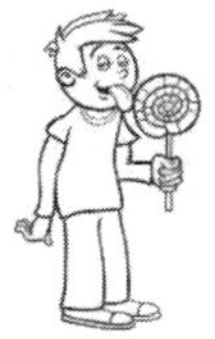

The Gustatory System and the Olfactory System

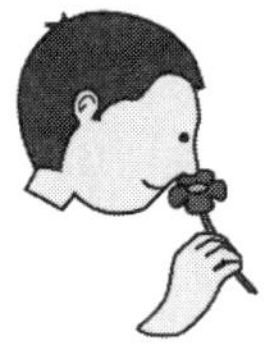

The following systems are those that affect an individual's sense of taste and smell. Many children with autism have extremely sensitive reactions to the smell and textures of the foods they eat. Some children will become nauseous at just the thought of putting a soft textured food in their mouths. Others often smell something in food that makes it inedible for them. This can be a "wiring issue" in the brain, rather than a behaviour issue. Overly strong responses to smells and tastes in persons with autism is research based.

Information regarding the olfactory and gustatory systems may seem somewhat out of place in an educational resource. However, food is part of our social relationships. At school students may celebrate birthdays or holidays together. They often eat snacks and lunch as a group. Educators that understand the whole story of sensory dysfunction will be far more patient and less likely to judge a child's eating habits – or a parent's food choices for their child!

Sometimes, teachers who have a good relationship with a student may be able to play a role in alleviating some eating issues. I remember teaching a young teen who would not drink water. The first time he had a sip, he threw up. But, knowing that water is critical in health, our team began implementing a system - three times a day this young man had to touch his lips to water. It was on his visual schedule. Within weeks we increased his contact with water as his tolerance increased. I am proud to say that within a year this student drinks water willingly.

As a teacher, I have had more luck introducing new foods and tolerance for clothes than the parents of some of our students have experienced. In fact, with parent's approval and with the input of Occupational Therapists and Speech and Language Therapists our team helped children break through some of their autism sensitivities. I believe our success is due, in part, to creating an environment where the child is accustomed to learning new skills and by breaking the typical response pattern created unwittingly at home.

Let me explain. Parents in their hectic and often frustrated daily lives can inadvertently reinforce unwanted responses in their children. Upon further investigation, our team learned that the boy who did not drink water was often given chocolate milk or Pepsi when he threw up. I might throw up too, if I knew I would be rewarded. A boy who would not eat any vegetables at all would cry out in a heart -wrenching wail, "Mommmy!" Naturally, his mom discontinued introducing the new food.

Another boy, who would refuse any food other than dill pickle chips and dill pickles, would scream uncontrollably until he received dill pickle chips. When we look at what happens immediately after the behaviour (gag, vomit, cry) we see what might be reinforcing and maintaining unwanted or negative behaviour. These behaviours can be changed by modifying our response. This means, no soda after vomiting and not giving in because of whining and sulking.

Healthy eating has a direct impact on learning. Teachers are not able to magically sustain the child's attention while the blood sugar levels spike and dive due to lunches filled with sugary, high carbohydrate snacks. Food which feeds the brain is essential for all students but it is sometimes more challenging for a student with strong sensory issues. Patience and perseverance will pay off in time when we keep providing healthy food. Behaviours will change with consistent intervention over time.

Choose your battles wisely. Forcing a child to eat foods that cause him to gag will only create tension and strain in your relationship with the child. These are not the kind of children that parents or teachers can leave at the table until they finish the food on their plate. Kids with autism have incredible associative memories. Do you want to be remembered as the one who forced him to eat something that he couldn't tolerate?

Gustatory System	**HYPER Sensitive**	**HYPO Sensitive**
This is the system in our body that receives information through his mouth.	Gags, refuses to eat certain foods Restricted eating habits May not enjoy soda drinks Dislikes brushing teeth Tastes food with tip of tongue Takes tiny bites of food or chews for a long time	Tastes or licks EVERYTHING! Enjoys strong tastes (spicy) Constantly seeks food (may raid the kitchen at all hours of the day!) May chew on non- edible items

Olfactory System	HYPER Sensitive	HYPO Sensitive
This is the system in our body that receives information through the nose.	Avoids rooms in the house, or places that "smell bad" (according to his or her own perception) Refuses to eat certain foods based on smell Difficulties with toileting due to the smells associated with washrooms Wears the same outfit repeatedly Complains loudly that something smells (appears rude)	Smears bowel movements Sniffs food and just about everything else Pica (eats objects that are not edible) Licks objects and food

I will close the section on sensory challenges with a personal experience to illustrate the positive and liberating impact that acknowledging and facilitating sensory support can make in an individual's life. When he was *finally* invited to a birthday party (at age ten), we were very concerned that Kieran might experience a meltdown given all of the sounds, smells and loud kids. The day before the party we visited his friend's home and discussed some potential problems with the host parent. She could not have been more warm and eager to make this a good experience. Kieran and the host agreed upon a spot where he could go when he felt that he was beginning to overload. We discussed the 'itinerary' of the party and surveyed the 'safe' places and people.

With my stomach in my throat I left to pick him up from the party. The birthday boy's mom was pleased to announce that like all of the partygoers, Kieran had enjoyed the festivities. Just before the cake and singing, Kieran quietly asked her if he could go to the quiet spot (which was a tree-house out in the yard). He came back to the gift opening and waited patiently while his friend opened the gifts. He was able to handle most of the party only because we had planned ahead for his own self - regulation. On the way home, Kieran reported proudly that the sounds were "starting to be wild in his head" he went to the tree house. This accommodation made it possible for our son to finally be a part of an activity for which he had longed. Interestingly, he and the birthday boy have been friends for 8 years. Love and respect goes a long way to building strong relationships.

The late, Stanley Greenspan, author of, *The Challenging Childl* (1995) used insightful analogies to help us understand what people experience when they cannot effectively process or interpret, sensory input:

- Every time someone touches you, it feels like they are rubbing sandpaper on your skin

- You feel like someone has given you a shot of Novocain in your backside so you can't feel if you were sitting in the middle of your chair and you fall off 3 times while reading this book
- You want to write something down but it takes you at least 5 seconds to form each letter. You can see the letter in your head, but your hand will not go in the right direction to write it.
- People's whispers sound like they are yelling

What follows is Greenspan's car analogy. It illustrates the frustration of living with a sensory system that does not work efficiently.

"Imagine driving a car that isn't working well. When you step on the gas the car sometimes lurches forward and sometimes doesn't respond. When you blow the horn it sounds blaring. The brakes sometimes slow the car, but not always. The blinkers work occasionally, the steering is erratic, and the speedometer is inaccurate. You are engaged in a constant struggle to keep the car on the road, and it is difficult to concentrate on anything else."(Greenspan 1995 p.4)

A summary of significant sensory characteristics that impact learning and relationships:

- Visual channel may be the most effective medium for attention and learning
- Might enjoy being squeezed or squished, swinging, jumping (a trampoline saved our sanity!)
- May overreact to being touched or hugged unless the individual initiates the touch
- Might appear to be deaf to some sounds (his name being called) but hypersensitive to other sounds (an airplane far in the distance)
- Eating a restricted variety of foods (e.g., only french fries, Lily Dale Chicken, and/or refusal to eat pasta or meat)
- Appear to be fascinated by some visual stimuli, experiencing difficulty breaking his attention – ceiling fans, brick patterns, windmills in the garden
- May exhibit an extreme aversion to certain textures by screaming and/or avoidance (tags on clothing, polyester, seams on socks or clothes etc...)
- May appear insensitive to injuries that are painful (indifference to a deep cut)
- Insensitive to extreme temperatures (refuses to wear a coat in the cold winter months or insists on wearing sweatshirts in the hot summer months)
- Over sensitive to heat (wince when a warm blanket is placed on her, refuse to play outdoors on a sunny day)

- May have unusual fears of harmless things (houseflies, computer printers, fax machines etc...) and yet not be afraid of typical things (dark rooms, traffic, being lost)
- May withdraw, cry or exhibit challenging behaviour in environments that are visually or auditory chaotic (assemblies, amusement parks, cafeterias, school hallways)
- Licks, smells or rests face on cement, bricks, tile floors
- May need time to be alone or to escape; this is critical in the school environment

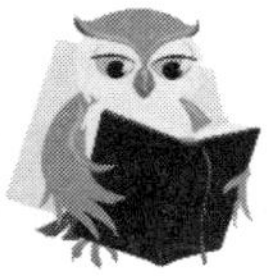

> ***"One of my sensory problems was hearing sensitivity, where certain loud noises, such as a school bell, hurt my ears. It sounded like a dentist drill going through my ears."***
>
> ***Temple Grandin 2006***

Beyond The Diagnostic Criteria

Cognitive Differences: The Trouble with Thinking

WARNING:

By the nature of their job, educators need to be economical with their time and energy. We tend want 'professional development' that can be put in place on Monday.' We need to be efficient - or we would get swallowed up in reading education and never have time or energy to implement what we learn. I need to warn you: the following section is larger and more detailed than the section on diagnostic criteria. It had to be. It is the 'stuff' that rarely gets to frontline educators and yet it is hugely critical teaching information. **Please do not do skip over it.** Reread it. Let it sink it and change the way you think about and intervene with students with autism.

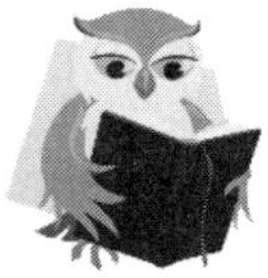

> ***"The essence of autism is in the mind, not in the behaviour."***
>
> ***Dr. Peter Vermeulen, 2012***

In the years since the first edition of this book was written, I have come to understand that the cognitive and neurological patterns in the autistic brain are far more significant to individuals with autism, their parents and teachers than I had ever fathomed. Given that the brain is the control center, it seems obvious that what happens in the brain, affects every aspect of human functioning. A traumatic brain injury drove that point home personally. Brain research in autism is changing the whole framework from which I approach, plan and organize supports for individuals and families with autism.

I do not pretend to understand the intricacies of the neurological and information processing differences in the autistic brain. Although, I admit I do have a compelling zeal to read everything I can get my hands on in this area. I study research with the eyes and mind of a teacher searching for clues as to how I can better understand and subsequently intervene and teach my students with autism.

In the first edition of this book, the current section focused on the impact of autism on the higher level cognitions and the resulting conscious thinking patterns. Since then, self- reports from well- known autistics such as Temple Grandin and researchers such as Peter Vermeulen, Nancy Minshew, Marcel Just, to name a few, have changed my understanding of autism's impact on the brain's lower level, perceptual processes. Differences in this area of the autistic brain result in differences in the unconscious perceptual patterns experienced by those with autism. Since both cognition and perception impact learning and living in the world, this section will first examine (to the degree possible in a book about IEPs) the differences in subconscious lower levels of information processing. Next, the differences in conscious, higher order cognitive processes will be the examined in order to give educators a better sense of how our students with autism think and perceive the world.

Thankfully, research on the neurology and functioning of the autistic brain is beginning to trickle down to the people on the front line: teachers, paraprofessionals and parents. It is an exciting time as we expand our understanding of autism. Because students with autism cannot choose the way their brains perceive and think about the world, (this is also true of neuro-typical persons) an increase in educators' understanding of autism should grow into an increase in respect, inclusion and appropriate support. I think educators can and should lead the way in modeling progressive thinking about supporting and honouring human differences.

Brain Differences and Complex Information Processing

Autism is better known and understood as a biological and neurological developmental disorder because it is the differences in the brain that create differences in language, communication, social interactions, cognition and behaviour. Information received from the senses travels to the brain and is processed through a series of interconnecting neural networks communicating with each other. Think of it as massiv e highway systems that transmit information throughout our brains. In brains with autism, some of the neural networks experience a disconnection that cause information to be processed differently. One area of the brain fails to communicate efficiently with another area when "long distance" integration needs to happen: during social interactions, reading and writing, for example (Minshew & Williams, 2007). When areas of the brain fail to coordinate efficiently, information is processed more slowly or inadequately. On the other hand, some 'short routes' (local) may be 'overly connected' (Grandin, 2013, p.31). Over-connectivity seems to be occurring in regions of the brain involved in visual processing (Supekar, *et al., 2013).* Researchers have also found that in some circumstances information is being processed in a different area of the brain than the same information would processed in a typical brain. It has also been well documented that, in the brains of individuals with ASD, there are structural differences in white matter volume (Williams & Minshew, 2010).

Each task we ask of a student, whether it is listening to a lecture, writing a report, participating in a group or solving a mathematical problem, requires a cognitive effort or load. We may think we have a sense of the magnitude of that load, but, the reality is that the brain requirement for each individual is highly individualized and dependent on many factors. Something that seems simple to us may in fact require a large amount of mental capacity on a particular student. Students use less mental effort (reducing the cognitive load) when they employ strategies such as categorization, selective attention, and automaticity. You have probably guessed that for students with autism, the very ways that could help reduce cognitive load are often impaired. In an autistic brain the innate and subconscious process of categorizing information coming from the senses does not function properly. Researcher, Nancy Minshew has likened the result to be analogous to 100 airplanes attempting to land at an airport simultaneously (Eltze, 2002).

When information is more simple and concrete the student with autism is able to process as efficiently as a student without autism. For example, reading word lists, computing simple calculations, mechanical reading are not challenging tasks for students with autism. However, information is processed with increasing **inefficiency** as the complexity of that information increases. (Williams et. al., 2006)This is critically important information for teachers.

What makes information more complex?

- The amount of information being presented
- Grammatical structure beyond simple sentences: sentences that include phrases and clauses complicate learning
- Intricate storylines, plots and themes
- Intricate or complicated visual scenes
- Time constraints (time tests, response times)
- Stress and anxiety (slows down thinking and processing)
- Multitasking (even doing two simple tasks simultaneously: taking notes and listening; listening to another's words while watching their facial expressions; chatting with a friend while walking and watching for traffic; making eye contact and listening to the teacher)
- Multifaceted motor movements (handwriting, tying shoes, dribbling a basketball, skipping)

Always keep in mind that, for a student with autism, what is complex is dependent on the individual and on the situation/context. Age and perceived intelligence are not fair indicators of what we should expect. We need to constantly consider what cognitive resources a student may be using. Then we can decide how much more complex we can make a task without causing cognitive overload (which may in turn produce shut down, emotional meltdown or behaviour challenges).

Information processing demands may be hidden in tasks that we might not realize. Nancy Minshew found that high functioning people with autism can understand long sentences as long as they were grammatically simple. But, if the same number of words were used in a different order, the level of comprehension decreased! Minshew learned that when there is a clause, the brain must process the meaning of the first part of the sentence and hold it in working memory, then process the meaning of the second part of the sentence, and then process the meaning of the first part in relation to the second part (Kana et. al., 2006). Consider for a moment the challenge it must be for someone with autism to process the language we use in daily life as it is fast paced and grammatically complex!

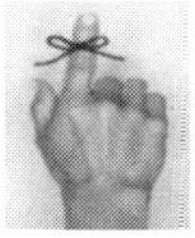

Memory and Information Processing In Autism

Impairments in memory are not part of the diagnostic criteria for autism and yet they are very much a part of the autism learning profile. We often assume a superior memory for those living with autism because they have a large capacity for remembering details and large amounts of unrelated data. But, working memory for complex information in both word and picture form is impaired in autism. Complexity is increased by adding to the volume of information or making complicated information. Impaired memory is especially noticeable if a child had to use an organizing strategy or notice an organizing strategy within the information to be remembered. It is as if the perceptual regions of the brain fails to tell the higher thinking and reasoning areas what is most important to pay attention to and the latter region fails to come up with an organizing strategy that would make remembering more effective. Functional neuroimaging (fMRI) is providing evidence that the memory difficulty in autism lies in "connectivity between perceptual and memory regions and differing information processing strategies" (Williams et. al., 2006).

Working memory is a construct that helps us hold on to information long enough to use it. Information isn't stored indefinitely in working memory; it is only there long enough to be played back while making use of it. Think of it as a 'sticky note' in our brain. Visual information comes to the 'visual spatial sketchpad' of working memory and helps students hold onto it for a brief time before it is lost. This specific process allows students to visualize something and keep it in their "mind's eye." Students use this skill to do math and to remember patterns, images and sequences of events. It helps them to remember over time where something is located once it is out of sight. Once they have sounded out words, visual working memory helps kids remember what those words look like so they can recognize them throughout the rest of a sentence.

Students who fail to "see" the inherent structure of a text or to use organizational strategies to help to remember information are demonstrating weak spatial working memory. Given that we tend to see autistic individuals as having a relative strength of visual memory, it seems odd that that visual spatial working memory can be a problem. Even visual information, such as a pictorial or social a scene will cause an overload in working memory when increased in the amount or the complexity.

Sounds and verbal instructions are briefly held in the verbal - auditory component of working memory. Anytime students are expected to follow a multi-step set of oral instructions, they are using these working memory skills. Auditory working memory helps kids hold on to the sounds letters make long enough to sound out new words. A student who is still sounding out words while reading is relying heavily on verbal working memory. This is very taxing to the working memory system and affects reading comprehension.

Not surprisingly, difficulties with working memory can wreak havoc on learning and academics. Complex subjects such as reading comprehension, mental arithmetic, and word problems rely on an effective working memory because they require various parts of the brain to communicate with each other quickly and efficiently. Even simple tasks such as copying from the board and navigating the hallways insist that we keep information in mind while we use it to get to where we are going. (Have you ever arrived in a room and forgot why you are there?) A child with low working memory capacity may find it hard to write sentences because by the time he finishes spelling the first few words, he's forgotten what he wanted to say next. Similarly, he has trouble with reading comprehension; while he's working hard to decode written words, he loses track of the overall "gist" of the text.

Even social functioning is impacted by inefficient working memory. Consider how much information comes to us simultaneously in any given moment that we share with another person. Body language, facial expressions, tone of voice, the physical environment and the emotional landscape send vast amounts of data to the brain. The visual and auditory working memory system is supposed to hold what is important so that the appropriate responses can be made. For an individual with autism, the 'load' will likely be too much and the result could be inappropriate or ill -timed responses, 'shut downs' or meltdowns.

Nancy Minshew makes the point that, "*If the brain does not, from the start, automatically identify and store key information that seriously impairs the capacity to interact, communicate and solve problems. Children with autism can be easily overwhelmed by the complex information in most everyday experiences*." She goes further to explain how these memory problems can affect behaviour: "*Typical people automatically notice and focus on what's important or relevant, but because people with autism focus on details instead, they can't recall or respond to what most people think is important* (Minshew, 2006).

Working memory challenges can certainly look a lot like behaviour problems. Does this student sound familiar?

- Abandons assignment midway through completion
- Forgets the second step of what he was supposed to do
- Needs incessant reminders to get back to the task at hand
- Fails to get started on a task
- In spite of the fact that it is an everyday routine, he fails to unpack his backpack and put his homework in the bin
- Cannot retell a story (in his own words) in an organized, sequential manner
- Has trouble doing math in his head

Given the challenges of information processing and memory impairments, it stands to reason that when we convey information to a person with autism it is crucial that we stick to the fewest words possible; we state the bottom line and provide visual back up. The length of our lesson will directly impact the degree to which a child with autism learns. Keep it short and to the point if you want it learned. In my role as a parent and a teacher, I have finally figured out that, for the child with autism, I need to state the bottom line succinctly. This, by the way, is not my strength! At the same time, providing a visual record of the bottom line and the steps and instructions gives a more permanent nature to our demands and eases the burden on working memory.

Working memory is not the only type of memory affected by autism. **Episodic memory**, a memory that is linked to a personal experience in a time and place, allows us to consciously travel back in our minds through time and recall or 'relive' an event. In your mind, I am sure you can recall an occasion you shared with a loved one. Perhaps, you recall pieces of the memory: a great meal, laughing hysterically over something, or maybe even the smell associated with the place. Persons with autism show a decreased ability in remembering the context and order of events or experiences in which they were a part. They tend to have fewer memories of past activities and relatively little memory of the feelings associated with the event (Bowler et al., 2000).

As we experience life, 'episodes' held in our memory allow us to draw from them the similarities, combine the "pieces" of the event, recall our preferences and create mental pictures of future episodes. Our episodic memory allows us to enter a new situation and figure out what to do because we remember a similar situation from our past. Recollection of past experiences provides the basis we need to negotiate peer interactions and relationships in the present. We are supposed to learn from our mistakes. Imagine not being able to access the emotional and contextual parts of those memories? Autobiographical memory of a past success can give us the confidence we need to take new risks. We are able to remember the fear, the effort and/or the feeling of achievement and use those memories to propel us forward. Despite an impaired episodic memory, individuals who live with autism have a strong associative memory and are more likely to remember the semantic details and facts of a previous situation. Semantic memory allows us to recall facts, definitions and information outside of ourselves. Consider how difficulties with episodic memory might impact a student's ability to relate a personal memory, write a journal entry or a personal narrative.

Perhaps the most detrimental result of an impaired episodic memory is its impact on learning. Students who 'remember' more about their learning experiences are more likely to schematize this information and show a higher level of understanding about the concepts (Herbert & Burt, 2004). Once again, we can see opportunities to schematize information might be lost for those living with autism.

As teachers, we need to know that, for students with autism, the learning process is enhanced when we make learning experiences memorable. We also know that students' interest in learning material is stimulated by real life, practical examples and they feel they learn better when material is presented in a more meaningful and relevant context. Given a poor episodic memory it is imperative that the learning environments and materials we use are explicitly connected to the life of the student with autism. This could mean connecting the learning to a strong interest or having the student use the skill in a real life context. If we don't teach the '*why*' of a skill, the chances are great that it won't even flash on a kid's radar. Why will I need this? Why does it matter? Our students with autism demand relevance. The more memorable and relevant we can make the learning activity, the greater quality and degree learning will be encoded in long term memory.

When we teach using hands on, experiential activities our students with autism will not intuitively be able to develop understanding of the concepts being taught to the same degree as students who do not have autism. However, this does not mean that our students with ASD cannot gain conceptual understanding through experiential learning, it simply means that they need explicit instruction within the experience. Children with autism learn much, much less from the environment.

Context Blindness

Problems with memory occur because the autistic brain inadequately uses context. In addition, reduced concepts and schemas leave the brain fewer options to access. Dr. Peter Vermeulen, an Autism Consultant and Lecturer at Autisme Centraal in Belgium has worked tirelessly to open typical minds to the minds of those with autism. His research on "context blindness" in autism and his book, *Autism as Context Blindness*, have dramatically changed the way I personally think about autism and more importantly, the way I teach autistic individuals.

A typical brain is wired with an innate ability to discover contextually relevant information and ignore contextually unimportant information. "*Context is what is going on in the environment, outside and inside our brain that influences our way of giving meaning to things*" (Vermeulen 2012, p.37). It can include anything within the mind: our ideas, knowledge, experiences, feelings (internal context). In addition, context can be anything outside of our mind in the physical and social world (external context) that influences how we perceive information coming to our senses (a stimulus) and what meaning we attach to it. Individuals with autism experience different thinking and cognition at least in part, because their brains are less sensitive to context .Subsequently, the way a student processes information (especially social information), develops concepts, understands communication, uses language and develops common sense and flexible thinking are impacted.

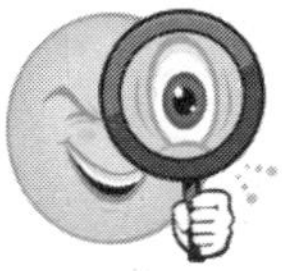

What Does This Mean for Teaching and Learning?

According to Vermeulen, the recognition of context happens subconsciously within 100 to 200 milliseconds - we don't have to focus our attention on what we already know and what the current circumstances tell us – our brain does that automatically. Dr.Vermeulen explains that we only notice details when we intentionally look for them. The fact that we miss a lot of details is probably a good thing because if we processed all the details it would be very tiring for the brain! Vermeulen uses the idea of 'seeing the forest for the trees' to illustrate how the non -autistic brain works. When we see a forest, without even being aware of the process, the lower processes in our brain perceive the essence of 'forestness' and our brain sends those perceptions to our higher cognitions. From there we use our conscious top down processes (thinking) and the information we know about forests from our mind notices the details from the physical world and we can consciously know we are seeing the details – the trees (Vermeulen, 2012, p. 50).

In contrast, people with autism see the details first and must do more conscious work to assemble the context or the whole situation. Given that context or the 'essence' of a situation works to focus attention on details that matter, it makes sense that those who do not have the benefit of using context tend to receive all the details.

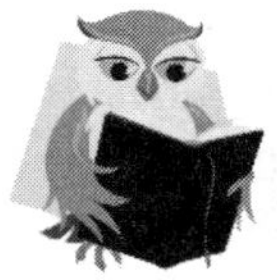

"When you see an object, it seems that you see it as an entire thing first, and only afterwards do its details follow on. But for people with autism, the details jump straight out at us first of all, and then only gradually, detail by detail, does the whole image float up into focus."

Naoki Higashida

Temple Grandin also sheds light on the difference in autistic thinking:

"Imagine if you had a thousand-piece jigsaw puzzle in a paper bag and you had no idea what the picture on the box is. When you start to put the puzzle together, you will be able to see what the picture is when it is approximately one-third or one-quarter of the way completed, When I solve the problem, it is not top-down and theory driven. Instead, I look at how all the little pieces fit together to form a bigger picture… I called this finding the basic principle. On everything in life, I was overwhelmed with a mass of details and I realized that I had to group them together and try to figure out unifying principles for masses of data." (Grandin, 2009)

In her book, *The Autistic Brain*, Temple explains that the 'bottom up' processing style means that she, and others like her, can see the trees in the proverbial forest far more acutely than the forest. She can see the trees in isolation. Grandin confirms Vermeulen's thinking that autistic people struggle to see the 'big picture' or the forest in this example (Grandin, 2012). As Temple points out, people with ASD recall a wealth of detailed information - but this is a sign of their failure to form schemata and categorize information as it comes to them from perception. This huge load of uncategorized information bogs down information processing, making it a slow and onerous process.

Without knowing a thing about context sensitivity, in his last year of high school, our son articulated an eye opening personal example of his challenge with context blindness. His English teacher informed us that he had been late in getting his chapter assignments handed in but he had performed reasonably well in terms of comprehension. Our first instinct was that he had been slacking off and my husband

and I were already planning which privileges he would lose, when he shocked us with a peek inside his thinking.

We asked him to lead us through the steps of how he would complete his novel study. His response was that he had had to read the whole novel before he could answer any questions in a chapter. Kieran explained that while listening to his classmates, he would wonder how they “just knew” what was going on in the book. He was astounded by the fact that even students who were least interested in the course were able to “have a clue” about what was going on in the novel. When probed about what he did to gain his own understanding of the novel he said that he had to work really hard to read the whole text so that he could go back and understand each chapter. Kieran could not see the essence, the theme or the gist automatically. On the other hand, his classmates were able to do so by reading the title, the back cover and listening to the teacher’s introduction to the book.

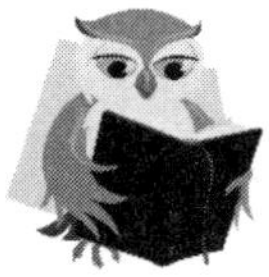

“In the blink of an eye we see the essence of a scene (the context) by a fast, subconscious transfer of info to the higher regions of the brain…when this scene recognition reaches our conscience we notice the details using top down processes which are slower and more conscious.”

Dr. Vermeulen (2012, p.51)

Concept Formation

Neuro-typical brains innately understand things conceptually, whereas an autistic brain does not (Minshew et. al., 2002). Instead, individuals with autism receive a whole lot of the details but the autistic brain disrupts the automatic process of categorization that happens in typical brains. The process of categorization is critically important for the development of conceptual understanding. The autistic brain has a great memory for details but because it does not automatically categorize information, thereby making information processing more time-consuming and slow (Williams et. al., 2006). The lack of spontaneous categorization of information also reduces the student’s ability to use what is learned experientially in new but similar situations.

A non- autistic brain detects resemblances while it subconsciously browses a collection of examples and/or a prototype (an average mental representation) of an object or an idea so that it is able to quickly and automatically decide if a new object ‘fits’ into a category. This is how we come to form concepts. We don’t have to consciously ‘think’ about it unless the concept is more abstract and cognitively demanding. On the other hand, in order to form a concept, a student with autism will have to use logic and memorized rules. Interestingly, children with autism (and even adults) tend to sort or categorize objects on a basic perceptual (size, colour or shape) level rather than a more conceptual and abstract level (things that are loud, items in the kitchen, games, and sports).

Very young children with autism may not even get the rules at this early stage; they may not associate meaning with anything. Teachers and parents may have to start from scratch in teaching a word that goes with an object for items that are known almost instinctively in other children. The world of a young child with autism is more fragmented and chaotic than we can ever imagine.

Using rules rather than conceptual understanding can lead to behaviour that seems odd or infuriating. After a year of begging, my husband and I succumbed to the pressure and allowed our son to have a pet rat. He was old enough and certainly mature enough to provide the care necessary. Fudge was a remarkably cute and gentle little addition to our family (in spite of his "ratness"). The pet store manager emphasized to Kieran how important it was that Fudge always had fresh water.

Kieran was a doting rat owner. He took good care of Fudge, played with the little guy and loved him dearly. But, for some reason, the little critter did not thrive. His death came as a shock to all of us – until we began asking questions. It turns out that one should never assume that a child with autism understands the concept that living things require *more* than water. Food perhaps might have saved Fudge's life! Our son faithfully followed the rules that were explicitly stated to him but he lacked a deeper, intuitive understanding of the essentials of life. It was years later when he approached us and abruptly asked if he had killed Fudge. The concept came – a little too late for Fudge.

As the story above illustrates, conceptual understanding develops when details come together as a cohesive whole. Contextual sensitivity helps our brains to pick out the important details and ignore those that will not aid in providing meaning. A very rudimentary explanation of how we use context to organize our thinking and our behaviour is illustrated in a shopping experience. We use context when shopping in Walmart™, for example. If I need to purchase shampoo, I use what I know about shampoo (internal context) and what I see in the physical environment of Walmart (external context) to find what I need. I know that my hair is colour treated (there goes my secret) and I remember that I don't like the results when I use an "all in one" shampoo and conditioner. Based on my internal knowledge and opinions I have a sense of what type of product I want to buy and where I would look for it.

I know that shampoo fits in the hygiene category. I use external context by noticing the sign displays in Walmart and I know to go to the Beauty and Hygiene area of the store. I even know from experience that it tends to be on my right when I enter the store. (In fact, I feel lost when the store layout differs from our store in my hometown). Within this section, I am able to use the signage to guide me to shampoo and then begins the task of scanning the shelves and pinpointing the one I want. I do not waste my time in the electronics department or the pet aisle. Consider also, how much more time consuming it would be to locate shampoo in a store that is unknown to you with signage in another language. The task is not impossible, but it will take more of a conscious effort to complete the shopping task. Context plays a significant role in our lives without us being conscious of it.

Like our knowledge (and Walmart), stories are built on a conceptual framework consisting of an internal structure and schemata: characters, plot, climax, theme and so on. Readers with autism will not be wired to 'see' the inherent structure. They are most likely to recall a wide range of details that are not necessarily the most relevant details that pertain to the main idea. This will make it difficult to tell and write stories and to relate their own personal experiences as a coherent narrative unless they are given explicit and visual support. A teacher may also notice that a student with autism tends to include every detail in what is supposed to be a summarizing task. The importance of using graphic story board organizers and teaching narrative skills cannot be understated. "Children need narrative skills for social and academic success (Franke & Dunn, 2011, p.3).

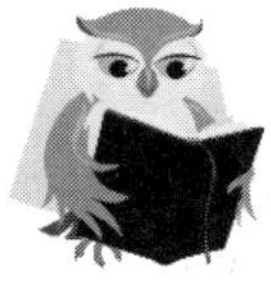

> **"Context helps us to know what to expect, recognize and finds things quickly, where to focus our attention and what to ignore and explains things that are not directly clear or understandable."**
>
> **Dr. Vermeulen, 2012, p. 85**

Students with autism often demonstrate **a literal understanding of language** and communication. Literal statements are our peek into the way an autistic mind derives meaning without context. Absolute meanings are assigned to objects, events or situations at least in part because the brain is not sensitive to context; it goes with what it already knows. But, that kind of thinking leaves our students incapable attaching a new meaning to concepts, words, actions and language resulting in inflexible and rigid thinking. Fixed meanings and one to one relationships devoid of context can lead to humorous situations. When he was ten years old, our son found it funny that our town had a place to wash coins: a 'coin laundry.' A teacher who has a 'stomach bug' or a 'frog' in his throat may create a frightening notion for a student with autism.

One of my favourite stories was shared by Dr. Rita Jordan, professor and Autism consultant at the 2003 Geneva Centre for Autism International Symposium. She told the story a student with autism who, upon seeing a squirrel on a garbage can, remarked, "*Oh look! Someone has thrown away a perfectly good squirrel!*" Anecdotes can be pretty funny but they also illustrate what the world seems like for those with autism: filled with isolated details, decontextualized meanings and lack of predictability. In familiar situations individuals with autism don't struggle with context because they have learned routines and they know what to expect. However, if we change something in the routine or situation confusion and unpredictability result because the autistic brain does not pick up on the context effectively to fill in the blanks or create a clear situation. "*Context helps us to know what to expect, recognize and finds things quickly, where to focus our attention and what to ignore and explains things that are not directly clear or understandable*" (Vermeulen, 2012, p.85).

Context and Communication

Not surprisingly, the ability to use context unconsciously, at super speeds, impacts our ability to communicate meaningfully. Individuals with autism can have a good vocabulary; they know the meanings of words (dictionary definitions) but are less able to use context to adapt word meanings to the real world use of them. The autistic brain tends to get stuck on the first meaning learned when words have multiple meanings.

High functioning students with autism can read single words, match them to pictures, and put words into concrete categories.

However, to read words, individuals with autism do not use context to the same degree as a neuro-typical reader. In fact, a reader with autism must process words more consciously and thus it takes more cognitive effort. This explains why our students with autism need more processing time in reading. According to Dr. Vermeulen, a non - autistic brain uses context within the first hundredths of milliseconds of information processing!

It doesn't help that our communication is rarely straightforward. The words, sentences, and phrases we use can have a multitude of meanings depending on the context. Consider the following statements and notice that there is more than one way to interpret the text.

My coffee is hot. (temperature)
The girl is my class in hot. (appearance)
This thai food is hot. (spicy)

"Hot" is a pretty simple word that can mean different things!

Think about these phrases:

"Get out!" This could be interpreted literally OR it could be an informal way of showing shock or surprise)

"We put our dog down." Again, this might relate to the action of placing your dog down on a surface OR it could refer to the death of a beloved pet!

The meaning we choose has everything to do with the context of the situation.

Considering that the autistic brain tends to assign absolute meanings to events, language and concepts it is really no wonder that confusion and atypical responses are often heard.

"Would you like to come in for coffee?"

Consider how quickly your brain reads between the lines of this statement given different contexts:

1. Two friends arrive at an apartment after shopping.
2. A man and a woman arrive at an apartment after having dinner together.

The invitation has different connotations or meanings depending on the context. To be clear, individuals with autism do not automatically look at the context and adjust the meaning accordingly.

The same is true for words that have many meanings, such as, in the case of homographs, homonyms and homophones. Because they do not automatically use context, these individuals have more difficulty knowing which meaning, pronunciation and spelling to use.

Homographs: words that are spelled the same but a different meaning and/or a different pronunciation (read, bass, lead, do, bow, minute, fine, row)

Homonyms: words that are spelled and pronounced the same but have different meanings (bear, cool, fast, bank, plant, glasses)

Homophones: words that sound the same, are spelled differently and have different meanings (sail/sale, mall/ maul, so/sew, seem/seam (when hearing the word, the context must be used to spell it correctly)

Problems with pronoun reversals are common in children and some adults with autism. Pronouns are referential words rather than absolute words. "I" can be "me" but "I" can also be "you", right? It all depends on the situation. One woman reported using "you" and sometimes "they" or "we" when she meant to say "I" or "me". Communicating with meaning is cognitive work for folks with autism.

Context and Social Relationships

The complementary theories of context blindness and theory of mind offer parents and educators insight into why social interactions and social thinking can be impacted by autism. Peter Vermeulen explains in his book:

Context plays an important role in emotional and social intelligence:

- *It activates our ability to empathize*
- *Helps us focus our attention on socially important info so we can decode facial expressions and body language*
- *Clarifies unclear body language and ambiguous facial expressions*
- *Gives us clues about the thoughts and feelings of others and gives us tips on how to respond to those thoughts and feelings*
  (Vermeulen, 2012, p. 166)

People with autism are able to empathize and they are able to recognize basic emotions in others but they tend to reason using intellect rather than emotion. The autistic brain is not built for emotional reasoning as is the neuro-typical brain. Thus, it is far less likely to attach emotional meanings to actions, words and body language. As they mature, folks with autism will likely be able to read the facial expression and even the mental states of others. Difficulties arise in knowing *why* someone might be feeling the way they do. What is causing an emotion? What is the other person thinking? What does the person know? What does he/she want? These are the crux of the problem in autistic social thinking. A typical brain is wired to automatically and even unconsciously think about the context (to pick up on the social – emotional cues, non- verbal language and so on) during social situations and interactions. The autistic brain, on the other hand, requires something to activate this kind of thinking. Remember that the brain with autism does not sort relevant and irrelevant stimuli automatically. It accepts *all* stimuli coming at it. It does not intuitively give social and emotional cues the attention needed to make ‘socially appropriate’ responses. Consider that a student with autism may be able to read the clear expression of anger on your face, know you are angry (because he has been taught) and yet, not make the connection between his or her actions and your response. We will need to make that connection for the student.

Facial expressions give us a window into a person’s thoughts, emotions and personality. According to researchers the context in which we see someone’s facial expression influences the way we scan that person’s face. People with autism observe a face differently: spending more time looking at less important parts of the face (ears, chin, hairline) and thus missing important contextual cues from the eyes and mouth (Vermeulen, 2012, p.24).

In addition to missing out on possible clues in a facial expression, individuals with autism do not use important external context clues (the where, what and who) to decipher the emotions or thoughts of another. External context can help to give meaning to non- verbal language. For example, tears streaming down a face carries many possible meanings.

Grief – if the context is a funeral
Joy – if the context is a wedding (unless the person crying is not happy about the wedding!)
Anger – if the context involves conflict and dissention

Even this list is too simplistic. The important point to keep in mind that facial expressions alone will often not give us enough information. We also use information coming from the voice, body language and we look at the facial expressions of others in proximity to help to find out more about emotions.

For this reason, teaching student with autism to simply identify emotions based on a static flashcard of a facial expression is ineffective in real life. Does a smile always portray happiness? Not a chance. A smile can be deceiving. It can be kind or mean spirited. Again, we cannot equate one facial expression with one meaning if we want to help our kids grow in social understanding.

One strategy that worked well with our son was to take many pictures of various people he knew well, in a specific context with a specific facial expression. For instance, a neighbor held a trophy and smiled broadly; a friend held a broken toy and frowned and so on. We found it useful to use quite extreme emotions as a start. How do we really demonstrate pride? Over time the discussions around these pictures led to guessing games about the emotions of others in malls, restaurants and social environments based on contextual cues. Another useful trick is to pause a movie at a point where a character is demonstrating an emotion and facial expression and talk about all the clues that exist regarding the way the character feels. At times, this game led to some hilarious ad lib lines that we would attach to each unsuspecting people engaged in heated interactions. At 18 years of age, and much to his sister’s annoyance, Kieran “gives a voice” to our two golden retrievers and I have to wonder if this stems from all our social emotional games when he was young!

People that have autism have to do a lot more conscious thinking about social situations, language, and communication than people who do not have the disorder because the autistic brain is wired differently. Individuals with autism are able to learn social do's and don'ts. They use rules to learn because they don't have the hardwiring required to make this social learning instinctual. But, rule based learning is problematic because it fails to take context into account.

Consider the rule, "Hitting a person is wrong." But is it still wrong if a mosquito has landed on the person? Is a congratulatory smack on the back unacceptable? Is a high five violent behaviour? Context directs the meaning attached to a behaviour. Interestingly, even if a child with autism can correctly determine if an action is wrong or not, when asked *why*, a child with autism is likely to explain the reason in an overly logical way or he will answer that he doesn't know. Often our students with autism fail to connect the rules and the mental states of others to the context. In the case of the mosquito attack, the victim is likely willing to endure a smack if it saves them from a swollen itchy arm. This may explain a whole host of recess complaints and breakdowns!

Successful social engagement requires that we communicate and act based on the context. Students with autism benefit from learning a script which outlines and explains a sequence of social interactions and social conventions necessary for a social situation (going to an assembly in the gym, greeting people in the school hallway, playing a board game and so on). However, our students will still need help adapting the script when the situation changes (going to a solemn service in the gym, greeting people in a line at the theatre, playing with more players). It is critical is that parents and educators help students with autism give meaning to different contexts by purposefully pointing out the relevant details and even more importantly, explaining how the details give us the meaning. We cannot leave this step to chance.

When dealing with **social –emotional problems**, a person with autism may be able to identify the details about a situation and may be able to recognize another's mental state but he or she will falter in making the connection between the emotion and the reasons for the emotion. What thoughts, concerns and expectations the other person may have remain in the dark for an autistic mind. Asking questions to discover underlying assumptions or providing an instruction (visual explanations using stick people and thought bubbles) may help to activate understanding.

No, your teacher glare is **not** likely going to produce a miraculous change in behaviour! To solve the problem will require a deliberate discussion about the context of the circumstances. Social problem solving for people with autism improves with age because they are able to gain a wider array of experiences to draw from. But it tends to be slower, more focused on the present and results in less effective solutions. Temple Grandin's explanation of some of her social learning offers educators an invaluable peek into the autistic perspective:

I did not know that eye movements had meaning until I read Mind Blindness by Simon Baron-Cohen. I had no idea that people communicated feelings with their eyes. I also did not know that people get all kinds of little emotional signals which transmit feelings. My understanding of this became clearer after I read Descartes' Error by Antonio

Damasio. From the book I learned that, in most people, information in memory is seamlessly linked with emotion. I have emotions which can be very strong when I am experiencing them, but information stored in memory can be scanned at will without emotion. It is like surfing the Internet of web pages in my mind.

Social relationships have been learned solely by intellect and use of my visualization skills. All my thoughts are in pictures, like videotapes in my imagination. When I encounter a new social situation I can scan my data banks for a similar situation that I can use as a model to guide me in the new situation. My data banks in social skills are also filled with news articles about diplomatic relationships between different countries and an archive of previous experiences. I use these scenarios to guide me in different situations. I then run videotapes in my imagination of all the possible ways to predict how the other person might act. It is all done using my visual mind. I have great difficulty with new social situations if I cannot recall a similar situation to use as a guide.
(Grandin, 2014)

The hardwiring of an autistic brain creates many social disadvantages:

- Inability to distinguish between behaviour that is accidental or intentional on the part of another individual
- Demonstrating inappropriate behaviour or poorly timed responses (laughing after everyone else has stopped laughing, interrupting another person and so on)
- Misunderstanding the meaning of statements or comments
- Force a student to focus on only one activity at a time (multi-tasking is too much)
- Cause a student to give up easily when trying to understand a complex process

To educators and classmates a student with autism may appear to be rude, selfish, obstinate, naïve and a poor sport. Compassion and openness to helping a student come from understanding that it is in fact, the autistic brain, that is creating these outward characteristics. To understand behaviour, we must understand the autistic brain.

Social thinking difficulties and insensitivity to context permeate reading comprehension skills for those with autism. These brain patterns help to explain why a student with ASD may struggle to understand a character's motivations or predict what a character will do based on these emotions and thoughts. Readers engage in a story by taking on the perspective of another person and they try to understand what characters are thinking and why they do what they do. Difficulty with this kind of thinking in real life makes it even more difficult to understand the thoughts and feelings behind what one character says or does and even more challenging to understand the interactions of various characters in literature. Students with autism may not be able to understand what is causing the emotions felt by a character. He or she may be unable to identify and understand deception within a story plot and the possible reasons for deception. To do so requires a student to understand and predict the emotions of the character based on the contextual emotional elements of the plot. It is imperative to keep in mind that for students with autism, the ability to comprehend the nuances of social interactions at a deeper level, more time and more explicit direction is a necessity.

Effective readers are able to apply what they know (world/background knowledge) to what they read, in order to gain a deeper understanding of text. The more readers know about a topic, the easier it is to connect the text with background knowledge. Students with autism tend to have a more limited background knowledge and schemata due to the impaired conceptual understanding (Bowler et. al., 2008).

A reduced range of background knowledge and subsequent failure to form concepts can be exacerbated because our students with ASD lack experiences. Withdrawing a student from activities due to "behaviour problems" will do far more damage to learning than one might expect. The fact that some individuals are less engaged in experiences that are not of particular interest to them will also dampen concept formation in areas of less interest. The autistic brain tends to hone in on certain areas of knowledge and experience rather than being open to a wide range of topics. Educators may notice a more restricted vocabulary, schemata and even social conversations for students with autism. A helpful analogy may be that given a smorgasbord of a wide variety of delicious food choices, the individual with autism might be totally enamored with one dish and it is as if no other food is available. Limiting oneself to one choice in turn limits the variety of experience with other tastes, textures and aromas.

In addition to a limited and highly focused background knowledge, a student with autism will not automatically use what they know and have learned to better understand the meaning of the text or to make connections. Even the common KWL charts (What do you Know? What do want to learn and what did you learn?), may be too open ended for our kids with ASD. Remember that an autistic brain fails to filter what is relevant and irrelevant. Parents and educators will have to be the context guides. We may need to use questioning to help focus attention on relevant information and build the bridge between the student's experience and the text.

Executive Function

Our kids with autism tend to struggle with executive function higher order thinking skills such as problem solving, abstract and hypothetical thinking and reasoning. A neuro-typical brain takes for granted its understanding of multiple representations, relationships, non-verbal language and so on. But, **abstract thinking** is problematic for student with autism because it involves reflecting on the attributes, ideas, situations and the relationships between situations and ideas that exist apart from the *here and now*. We will likely see deficits in a student's ability to understand less concrete ideas such as algebra, love, justice, irony and democracy. Students may have a hard time describing a concept in their own words and providing an explanation for the concept. Theories or concepts that describe relationships such as the food chain, cause and effect, group learning and such will be hard to grasp without explicit and concrete support.

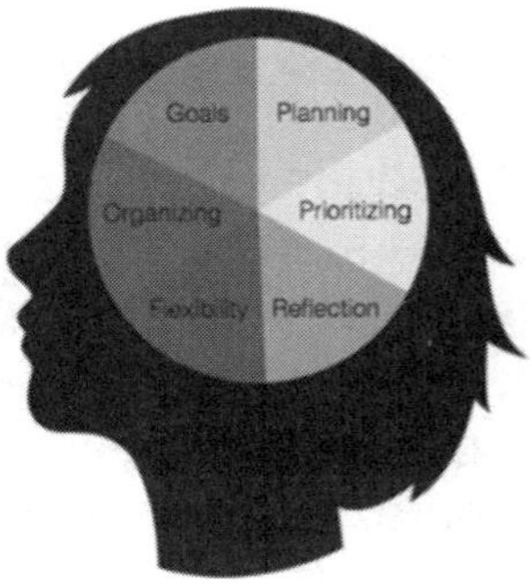

The concept of time can be very hard to grasp for a mind with autism (due once again, to neurological differences). The perception of time can be very fragmented and delayed. In a classroom a student may need more time to process verbal information because it takes a longer time to hear the words, figure out their context and prepare an appropriate answer. Remember, the brain regions don't communicate well with each other in autism. Time management is an important skill for all kids to learn, but, for a student with autism it is critical! Patience will be needed.

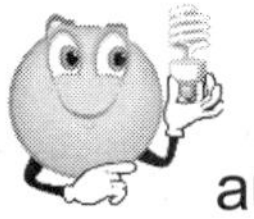

Critical thinking is a skill that poses significant challenge for individuals with autism. This shows itself in trouble with putting a series in sequence, making predictions or inferences, drawing conclusions, evaluating a concept or ideas, getting the main idea and making judgments about an event. This deficit in critical thinking really impacts the autistic student's comprehension of text and the ability to make decisions based on what they think the consequences may be. Critical thinking plays a key role in initiating and maintaining relationships, knowing when one is being teased or treated fairly. We use our ability to think critically when we make judgments about safe and healthy choices. Telling a child with autism to "think about what they did" is really quite a futile activity. Educators and parents will have to work through the whole problem or situation with visual representations if they want to make a lasting lesson out of the difficulty. Critical thinking skills, like so many others are best taught using graphic organizers and visual representations (webs, diagrams, software).

When students create visual diagrams they can use their visual strength to decide what is relevant and irrelevant, generate complex thoughts and draw connections between new ideas and make inferences. Diagrams and visual representations help students better articulate ideas and concepts, which aid in understanding the meaning of complex concepts. When asking open-ended questions ask students to create a web to think through the question, record research, structure thoughts. The process of creating the visual web or any graphic organizer, is by definition critical thinking.

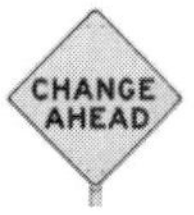

The ability of autistic people to concentrate on one thing at a time can be a blessing or a curse depending on the situation. If the student is involved in a project that he or she finds interesting, the level of engagement will be remarkable. But, if and when the need arises to change subjects or move to another classroom, the uglier side of focus may rear its head. **Set shifting** includes what we call transitions. Autism and transitions don't mix. Even high functioning individuals have trouble shifting their gaze and their attention from one thing to another.

Set shifting is required within tasks when a student needs to move from one problem to another. It occurs between tasks when a student must leave circle time and move to the snack table. Being able to accept "no" for an answer requires a shift in our minds, as does seeing someone else's point of view. Resistance to changes can appear to be rude, stubborn and disobedient behaviour when in fact they are just responses to the information the brain is providing. Rigid thinking can be caused by impaired set shifting and/or working memory problems. Definitely something to keep in mind in those situations when your blood pressure is elevating and you feel your own reasoning shutting down! The brain has a mind of its own; the student is not being willfully oppositional for the fun of it.

As we have learned, the autistic brain has trouble knowing which information is important enough to focus on. This is true in visual scenes, social situations, written text, verbal information and so on. In the classroom, a student with autism may find it distracting to shift their visual attention from the board to the teacher talking and back again, and as a result struggle to remember the lesson even if it is presented visually.

Weak inhibition skills, quite common in young children with autism, act to increase distractibility and deter from smooth transitions. Children with autism are able to understand rules such as wait your turn, first dinner, then dessert, but, they may not be able to control the impulse to overcome their desire. Direct teaching and rewarding impulse control is worth the investment of time, energy and patience as it will improve social relations, learning, and transitional changes.

Many teachers recognize early on that **planning skills** are often impaired in kids with autism. In order to plan efficiently, we need to have a goal in mind, know what steps we need to take, in a logical order. We also have to keep our attention focused on the steps and the goal and notice when we are straying off task (self -monitoring). Children with autism do not develop the components of planning as intuitively and flexibly as typical children. They may adhere to a strict script outlining how things should be done and failing to adapt when the need arises. When new players are added to a game, or a resource is unavailable plans need to change. Unfortunately, for a student with autism, set shifting, working memory and planning are not well developed and life can become very chaotic quickly.

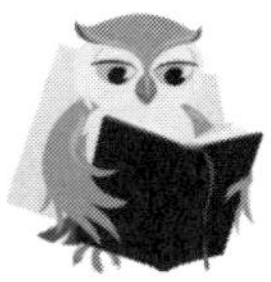

> ***"Without appropriate support, the child with ASD may feel he is drowning in a million sub tasks. Many of us have trouble prioritizing and organizing tasks."***
>
> **Dr. Stephen Shore**

My concern in outlining many of the deficit areas throughout the book is that somehow the reader will adopt a deficit mentality. This would be far from my intention. I strongly believe that the processing style of those with autism is different but invaluable in our world. We would not be where we are as a society if we did not have brains that think differently. The bottom line, I believe, is that educators and parents need to be aware of the differences in order to provide support for the learning process and foster an attitude of respect and understanding for differences.

Most people on the spectrum process things analytically based on facts and details. Emotional and situational context does not play a strong role in giving meaning to an event. This is most likely due to a lack of context sensitivity and problems with connectivity between brain regions. On the other hand, a non-autistic person tends to remember the emotional meaning and contextual details (episodic memory) of the event. Over time, we will probably forget the factual details of the event but hold onto the overall emotional meaning the event had for us. My wedding day memories consist of some details but what is the most strong is the memory of how I felt that day. My excitement and deep happiness of that day have had a lasting effect on my marriage because I can consciously 'go back' and remember the feelings associated with the event. The emotional context holds the memory and gives it meaning.

It is not that folks with autism don't remember strong emotions; it is more likely that a strong emotion such as joy, pride, or pain will be remembered in an intellectual and factual way. This way of thinking can lead non autistic people to assume that the responses of a person with autism are rude or inappropriate because we attach an emotional meaning to them. It is very likely that an emotional meaning or inference was not there in the first place; literal meaning is more likely. On the flip side, individuals with autism must have a hard time understanding why non autistic people don't just say what they mean.

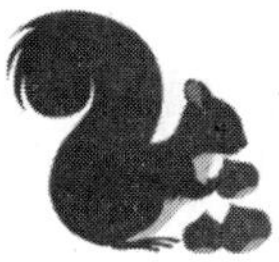

Cognitive Challenges in a Nutshell:

- Delayed information processing
- Concrete thinker and visual learner
- Absolute meanings result in literal understanding and rigid, inflexible thinking
- Impaired concept formation
- Insensitivity to what is important in the context
- Poor working memory for complex material
- Poor episodic memory
- Strong rote memory and associative memory
- Difficulty with abstract thinking, critical thinking, problem solving, time management and set shifting

Different Ways of Thinking

Keenly interested in brain differences within autism, Temple Grandin proposes that people with autism are "specialist thinkers." While autistic brains most likely share the ability to pick out details, hold vast amounts of information in long term memory and make strong associations, the way that these strengths are utilized differs amongst autistic individuals. Grandin explains that, like herself, there are individuals with autism that are "photo-realistic visual thinkers." She describes her thoughts as photographs of real objects that she has experienced.

In school, geometry and trigonometry could be converted to pictures in her mind but algebra was very hard for Temple because it could not be visualized. Visual thinking was Temple's strength and as such, it was developed into a highly rewarding career and life passion. She has revolutionized livestock handling by using her ability to see the world in a different way to develop a deeper understanding of animal behaviour.

Grandin suggests that students with a visual thinking brain might enjoy hands on activities, building with Lego, painting, cooking, wood working and sewing. Visual thinking kids may want to create things that look like the objects that they see in their mind's eye. Algebra and other math may be very challenging for these thinkers as it cannot be visualized.

Grandin points out that not all visual thinkers see realistic photographs or videos in their mind. Grandin's thinking begins with a still image which she is able to visualize from different perspectives. She is able to move her mind's eye around the image because she is an "object visual thinker." On the other hand, there are visual thinkers with autism that are pattern thinkers who are able to spatially visualize patterns (Grandin, 2013).

Temple Grandin hypothesizes that pattern thinking is a third type of autistic thinking. Unlike herself, this category of thinking involves more abstract thinking; patterns and relationships between numbers make these folks better at math and music. Worth reading are Daniel Tammet's book *Born on a Blue Day* (Tammet, 2006) and Jerry Newport's book *Mozart and the Whale* (Newport et al. 2007) as they describe pattern thinking in ways that are inspiring and intriguing. Grandin explains that pattern thinkers may struggle with reading and writing. Like object visual thinkers, they be drawn to constructing things, but, their brains are attracted to the way the parts of an image are put together, rather than creating something from a picture in the mind. According to Grandin, pattern thinkers see patterns earlier than others. They are usually good at math and music. Expert chess players see patterns and know what to do before it is their turn to move. Daniel Tammet used patterns to learn many new languages. Writing computer code, fashioning origami, solving crosswords and Sudoku puzzles are most likely products of pattern thinkers (Grandin, 2013).

The third type of autistic thinking described by Grandin is word fact thinking or verbal thinking. These individuals have a huge memory for verbal facts on all kinds of things such as horses, World War I and sports. They might love to make lists, record copious notes on their favourite topic and memorize things such as bus schedules and routes. Some individuals with autism have exceptional verbal reasoning skills and an ability to use language very precisely. According to Grandin, word fact thinkers might do surprisingly well in written assignments (given a structured organizer). Filing, record keeping and researching may be areas of strength. On the other hand, drawing and other visual thinking skills may be areas of weakness.

Far from comprehensive, the information on differences in autistic thinking is intended to be a starting point for educators and parents who are looking for ways to enhance their own and their child's awareness and understanding of strengths and weaknesses. I strongly encourage educators to read autobiographical information on individuals living with autism as an authentic way to deepen understanding and empathy. Appendix H is a list of people with autism who have inspired me personally and professionally.

Teachers are well aware of the diversity of learners. We know that most likely, brains consist of a mixture of thinking patterns. Autistic thinking is no different. Temple's growing understanding of the diversity of the autistic brain will hopefully widen our own view of the learning profiles of students with autism. The more we tune into individual thinking patterns, the better we should be at choosing the most effective teaching strategies and supports for a given child.

Motor Differences

While they are not considered in the diagnostic criteria, motor differences are prevalent in autism. Researchers like Megan MacDonald, who is an expert on the movement skills of children with autism, are finding a direct relationship between motor skill deficiencies and the severity of the symptoms of autism spectrum disorder in very young children.

Doctors Claudia List Hilton and John Constantino of the Washington University School of Medicine in St. Louis, affirm that children with autism often have problems developing motor skills, such as running, throwing a ball or even learning how to write. The study showed that the lower the level of motor proficiency in children with an autism, the greater the degree of social impairment and severity of the disorder (Hilton et. al., 2012). Given these results it makes sense that incorporating fine and gross motor skill development into early interventions and educational planning could improve IQ, language, play skills and independent functioning and self-esteem for children with autism.

Teachers might see:

- Poor handwriting (and subsequent low output of writing)
- Deficit in athletic skills and visual motor integration
- Awkward gait in walk and running
- Balance difficulties
- Poor motor coordination (prone to accidents, clumsy)
- Deficient fine motor skills (fasteners, handwriting, colouring, picking up small items, cutting with scissors)
- Difficulty starting and stopping actions (may need physical or verbal prompts)
- Unusual body postures, facial expressions stiffness of posture

Emotions and Anxiety

Considering that individuals with autism experience a variety of unusual sensory challenges and the language areas in the brain often leave folks unable to interpret or explain what is upsetting them, it is no wonder that anxiety levels are amplified. Add to that challenge a difficulty understanding and managing their own emotions and interpreting the non- verbal language and emotional nuances of others in a school filled with children and adults interacting at break neck speed. Living with a brain that insists on sameness, singular meanings and routine in a world that is unpredictable and chaotic at the best of times, must be a daily feat.

As we have seen in the previous cognition section, the brain of an individual with autism does not filter incoming stimuli well. In fact, the amygdala is ultra-quick to speed dial our emotions (without our conscious approval) to alert the body of immediate danger. This is normally a good thing. But, in a brain with autism, the frontal cortex (reasoning area) of the brain fails to do its job of determining whether the emergency is really a threat.

The result is that an individual is emotionally hijacked by things that would normally not be deemed, by the thinking brain, as real danger: house flies, the hand dryer sound, a touch on the arm and so on. We really shouldn't be surprised that anxiety and emotional overload play a leading role in the life of many individuals with autism. And we certainly should not be condemning such reactions!

On the other hand, it is surprising - and sad - that many times, educators and parents will claim that little Johnny is not anxious. They might argue that he is being stubborn and he just doesn't want to do his work, or participate. Perhaps Johnny cries because he is just really sensitive? It must be that his mother babies him too much! Not true. Behaviours exhibited by a child with autism stem from an underlying sense of anxiety and a brain that thinks differently. A neon sign doesn't flash over an individual's head announcing: "Be gentle, ANXIOUS PERSON DUE TO BRAIN DIFFEENCES below." I wish it did. At least then, we would have no choice but to address anxiety directly and compassionately.

What perhaps worried me the most as we raised our son, was his low self-esteem and an underlying sadness that showed itself most often at bedtime when he would say his prayers. He was lonely. He prayed for a friend. Like so many other children with higher functioning autism, Kieran was aware that he was different. He knew that he made others upset when he had a tantrum. He had difficulty identifying and expressing the emotions he felt. Throughout his elementary school years, what made the most difference was not that his teachers and principals had an expert knowledge of autism. It was their genuine love and concern for who he was as a person that drove their search for his positive qualities and gifts rather than focusing on his deficits. His best educators recognized where he needed support and seamlessly wove it into daily programming. Kieran instinctively knew when he was valued and he thrived emotionally in those classes.

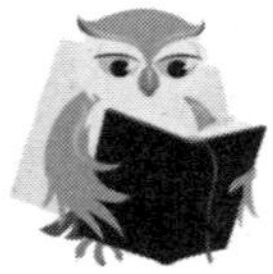

"When the anger is intense, the person with Asperger's syndrome may be in a 'blind rage' and unable to see the signals indicating that it would be appropriate to stop. Feelings of anger can also be in response in situations where we would expect other emotions. I have noted that sadness may be expressed as anger."

Tony Attwood (2008, p.143)

How Do I Teach This Kid?

Children with autism do not come to school to be cured. In fact, I don't believe they come to school to learn to be less autistic. If you are not sure whether you believe me, ask yourself if you expect that somehow your teaching will make a blind student less blind? A student with cerebral palsy less affected? I would like to suggest that our kids with autism just need to learn and grow into the person they were created to be. Like physically and visually disabled students, our autistic students will need different supports than other students in order to access the curriculum. They will probably need additional "curriculum" to facilitate development of individual potential. If we want our students to develop intellectually, emotionally and socially, we have to direct more focus on how we can create environments and learning tasks that stimulate personal growth and simultaneously mitigate anxiety. Reflecting on the way we relate to the student will go a long way to motivate learning. We simply cannot ignore or diminish the role anxiety and self -esteem play in any of our students. All humans need to feel loveable and worthy.

Experience and science have taught me some key principles underlying the creation of autism friendly classrooms and schools.

Acknowledge that the only autism experts are those living with autism

The more we learn about autism, the more we know that, we don't know much. We may spout the adage, "If you know *one* person with autism, you know *one* person with autism." But, I fear we continue to make assumptions (sometimes subconsciously) about an individual's strengths and weakness when we depend too heavily on textbook descriptions of autism or our own experience with other autistic students. I fear we can make dangerous assumptions based on what we think is a student's level of intellectual functioning and level of language. Yes, we have to rely on commonalities in autism if we are to keep up with the demands of teaching many learners with diverse needs in a classroom. But, it is essential – really, really critical - that we never allow our 'expertise' or assumptions to blind us from our genuine knowledge of the student as an individual. I recently had a teacher share her frustration about this very thing. A colleague had insisted that a student's diagnosis must be wrong – after all, the student had a great sense of humour and students with autism cannot have a sense of humour! Blanket statements are wrong. So wrong.

Challenge your own thinking

In writing a book about autism one of my biggest fears is that I would diminish the gifts of autism in the process of highlighting the needs associated with the disorder. In our role as service providers, parents and educators, we can get too caught up in what we believe needs "fixing." We may feel that we must repair all areas of weakness and impairment for the sake of the child. But, our children do not come to school to be "fixed." A person with autism is not "broken." Like any human being, there are certainly aspects of the person which require support and skill building. Creating autism friendly environments, capitalizing on strengths, teaching new skills and compensatory skills are all ways we serve our students with autism. But, at no point is our job to make them more like us, and less like themselves.

Raising a child with autism brought me face to face with this reality in a deeply personal revelation. At nine years old our son pointedly asked me, "If there was a pill that would cure autism would you give it to me?" Taking a minute to swallow the lump in my throat, I responded as I thought I should: "No I wouldn't."

My next words surprised me: "You wouldn't be <u>you</u>."

In that moment I knew without a doubt that I was speaking from the heart. Yes, autism is unbelievably draining on the emotions, finances, relationships, time and energy. But, with every fibre of my being I do not see an individual with autism (or any special need for that matter) as damaged goods. The gifts that autism has brought to my life through my son, my students and the families I work with have been far richer than I ever imagined. I am convinced that the way we choose to see the challenges will make all the difference in our own lives and in the lives of those we serve.

In her book, *The Autistic Brain*, Temple Grandin wisely notes, "*If even the experts can't stop thinking about what's wrong instead of what could be better, how can anyone expect the families dealing with autism on a daily basis to think differently*?"(Grandin, 2013, p.181)

I would humbly add, that given the focus on deficits by professionals, how are we to expect children with autism to view themselves as capable and skillful. What sense of self are we imparting?

Tony Attwood and Carol Gray, two internationally renowned autism specialists who have dedicated their lives to seeing the gifts of autism, have developed ingenious diagnostic criteria highlighting a more affirmative view of an autism diagnosis:

A. A qualitative advantage in social interaction, as manifested by a majority of the following: positive

(1) Peer relationships characterized by absolute loyalty and impeccable dependability
(2) Free of sexist, "age-ist", or culturalist biases, ability to regard others at "face value"
(3) Speaking one's mind irrespective of social context or adherence to personal beliefs
(4) Ability to pursue personal theory or perspective despite conflicting evidence
(5) Seeking an audience or friends capable of enthusiasm for unique interests and topics, consideration of details, spending time discussing a topic that may not be of primary interest
(6) Listening without continual judgment or assumption
(7) Interested primarily in significant contributions to conversation, preferring to avoid "ritualistic small talk" or socially trivial statements and superficial conversation
(8) Seeking sincere, positive, genuine friends with an unassuming sense of humour

B. Fluent in "Aspergese", a social language characterized by at least three of the following:

(1) A determination to seek the truth
(2) Conversation free of hidden meaning or agenda
(3) Advanced vocabulary and interest in words
(4) Fascination with word-based humour, such as puns
(5) Advanced use of pictorial metaphor

C. Cognitive skills characterized by at least four of the following:

(1) Strong preference for detail over gestalt
(2) Original, often unique perspective in problem solving
(3) Exceptional memory and/or recall of details often forgotten or disregarded by others, for example: names, dates schedules, routines
(4) Avid perseverance in gathering and cataloging information on a topic of interest
(5) Persistence of thought
(6) Encyclopedic or "CD-ROM" knowledge of one or more topics
(7) Knowledge of routines and a focused desire to maintain order and accuracy
(8) Clarity of values/decision making unaltered by political or financial factors

D. Additional possible features:

(1) Acute sensitivity to specific sensory experiences and stimuli, for example, hearing touch, vision and/or smell
(2) Strength in individual sports or games, particularly those involving endurance or visual accuracy, including rowing, swimming, bowling, chess
(3) "Social unsung hero" with trusting optimism: frequent victim of social weaknesses of others, while steadfast in the belief of the possibility of genuine friendship
(4) Increased probability over general population of attending university after high school
(5) Often take care of others outside the range of typical development

From: Discovery of "Aspie" Criteria © Carol Gray and Tony Attwood, 1999
As found at http://www.tonyattwood.com.au/index.htm, "Tony's Publications"

Develop Strengths

Early in our son's life, Temple Grandin impressed upon us the need to always develop Kieran's strengths. Our son is not savant. Only 10% of people with autism are. In a nutshell, developing strengths means taking the time to examine how a child's brain works and capitalize on the ways that it works well. Building on individual strengths to teach skills and practice concepts increases motivation and improves learning. Capitalize on strengths such as, matching, rote memory, spatial concepts and visual acuity (if those are a student's skills).

Expanding on an area of interest can be incredibly rewarding for teacher and student. Paula Kluth's book, *Just Give Him the Whale* (2008), is an exceptional resource providing many ideas about how to incorporate a student's passions into the classroom. Allowing students to doodle or draw in class and encouraging students to find materials of interest outside of their grade level are ways of building on strength. Honouring a person's gifts and valuing one's differences is far more effective (and fair) than focusing exclusively on deficits.

As educators, what we need to realize is that individuals with autism do not choose to think or perceive differently. They are, in fact, at the mercy of very real brain differences that impact the way they think, experience and view the world. It is incumbent on parents and educators to first, seek patterns of thinking and areas of interest and then capitalize on this knowledge. Search the school, online or in the community to find a mentor who shares a passion with a student. Allow the student to go beyond the grade level materials by linking the student with online resources or colleges or universities in pursuit of his or her interest. Do whatever it takes to nurture and expand the talent and/or interest in order to facilitate each student's personal growth and potential.

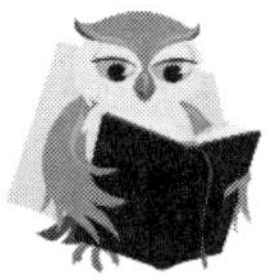

> ***"If we really want to prepare kids to participate in the mainstream of life, then you have to do more than accommodate their deficits. You have to figure out ways to exploit their strengths."***
>
> ***Temple Grandin (2013, p.184)***

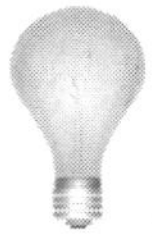

Dispose of the "That Doesn't Work, We Tried That" Garbage

Please allow a short rant here: Nothing slows progress and kills motivation more than a hopeless attitude. To be frank, this is a dead-end statement that makes me crazy! Yes, a strategy (such as visual supports) may have been tried for a period of time with no obvious results. However, it is very possible that it is time to try again! Kids with autism don't do well with change and perhaps more time was needed for the strategy to become a routine. More than likely the implementation of the strategy needs tweaking. In the case of visual supports, maybe words would be better than pictures. Maybe, the way that visuals were introduced was ineffectual. Is there a chance that the visual is not accessible or relevant for the student? There are many reasons why a strategy does not have the desired effect when it is used. This is precisely why it takes a team approach to raise a child with autism. My suggestion is that when we start to despair and frustration sets in, it is time to reach out, with an attitude of openness, for input from other professionals and parents. Change something in the way the strategy is being presented. Do whatever it takes. But do not quit trying. Model tenacity and perseverance for the student who needs those very qualities.

Decide that you **will** learn from this child

Kids with autism have taught me far more than I could ever hope to teach them! They keep us humble and always thinking ahead. Teachers constantly report to me that a student with autism fascinates them and leads them to think in ways they had never thought before. Yes, autism comes with challenges but what these students have to offer to those who look beyond the difficulties is perhaps richer than you can imagine.

Think inclusively

A whole book could be written on this subject, but, suffice it to say that students with autism **are** a valuable member of the classroom when we choose to think inclusively. Fear, doubt, overwhelm and lack of training can leave educators (and parents) seeing a child as a burden rather than a gift.

Consider comments such as, "*we are just glorified babysitters;*" "*our system should be spending more money on kids who will become something*;" and "*what are we supposed to do with that – isn't there somewhere else that student should be*?"

What if those comments were made about your child or a child you loved? Have we not evolved from the days of institutional dumping grounds? I certainly hope so. Children learn by what we ***do*** and by what we ***say***. Our society will become more inclusive and accepting as teachers model what it means to authentically include a child with special needs in the day to day activities and relationships of a classroom and a school. A child's peers will learn much from the way we speak to a child with autism and the way we respond to 'behaviour' and differences. The litmus test for every word, action and gesture should be, "Would this be acceptable if someone said or did it to a child that **I** love?" If not, don't.

Part of thinking inclusively is looking for ways that the student can participate meaningfully in class. Plan how the student will take part in activities throughout the day (see Appendix J: Assistive Technology Implementation Guide for ideas); catch yourself if you think he cannot do something. Instead, teach the skills or put the supports in place so that he is able to partake. Devise activities that enable him to share his special interests with classmates often.

Plan the tools needed and plan to **use** them

It is equally important that we teach the way that these kids learn! It is not enough to say that we have the tools available; the tools must be used consistently. A visual schedule is probably the most basic and yet the most critical tool that a student needs to support their activity at school and yet, too often they sit in a drawer somewhere and never see the light of day! It is just as ineffective to place a schedule in front of a student with autism or on the board, and expect the student to instinctively 'use' it. Having tools is not enough. We need to teach kids how to use the tools and we must expect them to be used consistently. Computers, software, sensory equipment, digital devices, augmentative communication devices and low tech tools such as graphic organizers, checklists and so on have no magic power until they are utilized consistently.

Make the Learning Environment Autism Friendly

I hate to sound 'preachy' but it is incumbent upon educators to organize the physical environment so that the student with autism is able to move calmly, purposefully and independently within the classroom. A great litmus test is to give a peer or a student instructions requiring him or her to access different areas of the classroom to carry out a task. Tasks might include putting homework in the homework bin, accessing a variety of supplies, choosing a book to read and so on. The 'guinea pig' should be able to carry out the task with no verbal prompts from you because the environment is set up to be very clear. Students with autism should know *how* and *where* to find items and replace things so that they can be as independent as possible. Thinking of movements and pathways ahead of time can also prevent problems that arise from distracting peers and/or activities while en route or trying to figure what to do.

Using the "Portrait of a Student" template in the Appendices, ask the student and parents to describe anything that might cause distress or discomfort (lighting, smells, noise and even specific persons). Plan a space for the student to work more quietly and/or with an aide. Think about an alternative to the chaos of recess. Perhaps, a quiet space, a student job or supervised club can be organized for at least some of the recess time. Recess is a nightmarish jungle for our kids because they are so ill-equipped to cope! Be sure to invest the time and energy into directly teaching and repeatedly practicing the routines and structures of the classroom and the school in order to build familiarity, safety and independence. This is good for all students!

Be prepared to work as a team

Children with autism most often come with a village of people. (We hope it is a productive village). By nature, autism is a multifaceted and complex disorder that demands many varieties of expertise. No teacher can do it alone. It is most helpful if you realize this ahead of time. Reach out for help. Accept help. Search for help. Autism has the potential to humble us and to expand our skill set all at the same time – if we work as a team.

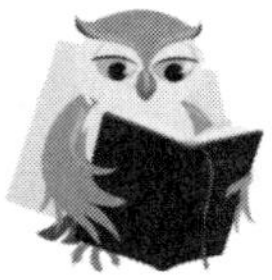

> ***"I believe autism is a marvelous occurrence of nature, not a tragic example of the human mind gone wrong. In many cases, autism can also be a kind of genius."***
>
> ***Jasmine Lee O'Neill***

A Closer Look at Autism Needs

While it is not within the scope of this book to provide a comprehensive resource of instructional targets that match the needs of students with Autism Spectrum Disorder, it is practical to outline some of the key points and strategies relating to some of the most common autism characteristics. Educators must use the needs identified by informal and formal assessments for each individual as a basis for developing an individual plan. The strategies that match a student's needs could be recorded in a learning profile such as the one included on the Appendix A: Portrait of a Student. The IEP does not include everything that you will do to facilitate learning for a student with autism.

Needs Associated with Social Communication

Given that language and social communication problems are hallmark symptoms of autism it is critical that we explicitly teach and practice social communication skills and concepts to our students who are on the spectrum. Communication and language activities targeted towards each individual's language and social deficits and strengths. Ideally, a speech pathologist should help to create programming goals and activities and monitor progress.

Consider these guidelines for Social Communication and Language training:

- ✓ Assess *how*, *why* and *where* the student communicates in order to develop meaningful goals – develop skills in real contexts where the child needs them
- ✓ Incorporate both receptive and expressive needs or strengths in the IEP
- ✓ Begin learning with concrete language and work towards more abstract language and use concrete aids/visuals whenever possible
- ✓ Even for higher functioning students, avoid long strings of information; use visual supports to aid comprehension and to check for understanding
- ✓ Create short, to the point social scripts and stories to activate context (teach what is expected socially and to explain social activities and events)
- ✓ Directly teach context clues and how to reference those around you—e.g., "if everyone else is lining up, you should be too"
- ✓ Set up situations in the classroom, school and community to practice social interaction skills that have been taught (partner interactions with scripts, negation (saying no), asking for help and so on)
- ✓ Include non- verbal language training (gestures, body language, facial expressions)
- ✓ Use peer buddies, commercial video models and video modelling to teach social thinking and skills

- ✓ Teach board games with one partner, using visual supports (wait cards, turn cards, simplified rules that are visually presented) - then expand to more than one partner
- ✓ Teach the student how to ask questions; play games where the student gets an opportunity to practice asking questions (I Spy, Guess Who? Go Fish)
- ✓ Create small lunch groups, perhaps with structured activities or topic boxes. Teach the group to pull a topic out of a box and have the students discuss things related to this topic, such as 'The most recent movie I saw was.....' This can be helpful for students who tend to talk about the same things all the time since it provides supports and motivation and the benefit of a visual reminder of what the topic is.) Retrieved from http://www.autismspeaks.org/sites/default/files/documents/family-services/improve_social.pdf
- ✓ Teach the *what* and the *how* of social skills AND the *where* and the *when*
- ✓ Ensure that we explain our actions and choose words carefully to avoid misunderstanding
- ✓ Teach narrative discourse skills (how to tell about past events, movies, stories, and so on in a cohesive sequential manner)
- ✓ Teach social pragmatic skills using visual supports/prompts and video modeling when possible (turn taking in conversation, varying topics/discussions, getting someone's attention, voice volume and so on)

Unlike typical students, those with autism do not instinctively know how to manage all of the complexities of human interaction. Students with autism need to be explicitly taught social – emotional skills. These skills should not be assumed to be "covered" in a series of isolated, one skill per worksheet types of programs. The following principles are essential for the student's social development:

- Teach with visual supports and structure (wait cards, 'My turn' cards, Social Stories ™ (Carol Gray), social scripts, simplified rules that are visually presented, explanations of specific context rules)
- Practice skills in natural context as much as possible (skills learned in isolation and outside of a real context will not be applied in a real context naturally)
- Provide a systematic, structured and long term approach that works on skills that are relevant to that particular student (social skills training is not a finite, packaged program)
- Use video models (commercial and homemade) whenever possible to teach real life and real time social thinking

- Enlist good social role models in social skills training groups and peer support as kids need to learn what is relevant to kids (especially slang and 'kid talk')

- Practice and reinforce very often and in different places, with different people until skills are used by the student in real life social situations without any prompts (mastered and generalized)

- Be prepared to review and discuss use of social learning skills over the long term to ensure the skills are maintained

- Include varying ages of peers in social group training

Utilizing the work Michelle Garcia Winner has done on Social Thinking™ led our son and many students to greater success and ease in social situations. Garcia Winner is a social skills expert that works on the front line and has written extensively on the deeper and more difficult aspects of social thinking that non-autistic people take for granted. Jed Baker is another favourite in the social communication arena.

The essential point is that without direct teaching and opportunities to practice skills, social communication skills will not magically develop for individuals with autism. Even higher functioning students who have no modifications in the regular curriculum need social communication programming. The need may not be obvious but it is very much a necessity. Autism always impacts the functioning of the areas of the brain that deal in the social realm.

Social skills training should follow the student's developmental level: teenaged boys and girls will likely need help with learning how to read the non- verbal language of the opposite sex and maintaining personal boundaries and relationships. As the mother of a teen with autism, I can tell you that many of our conversations are around dating, knowing when someone is flirting and developing the skill of social problem solving.

People take social understanding and the ability to read context clues for granted because the non-autistic brain is wired to do so subconsciously and quickly. We do not have to think about it very often. This is not true for people with autism and yet, it can be argued that it is more important than any other skill taught! We can have all of the academic honours that we are able to imagine, but without the ability to work with people and live in relation to them, happiness may be elusive.

Needs Associated with Language

For those with autism using language is far from a natural and instinctual process. In fact, it takes a lot of mental effort. We need to support the use and understanding of language in our students with autism by deliberately and systematically teaching the verbal and nonverbal aspects of language.

- ✓ Determine what means of communication a student will use to express ideas, needs and opinions. Use this means consistently and expect its use (see Augmentative Communication in resource list)
- ✓ Determine a student's receptive language needs using formal/informal assessments (make no assumptions without evidence)
- ✓ Directly teach and explain words with double meanings, metaphors and implied meanings
- ✓ Literal and concrete understanding of information necessitates increasing the comprehension of idioms, jokes, metaphors and all figurative language
- ✓ Nouns, prepositions and pronouns have to be introduced purposefully and as visually and concretely as possible (mixing up "I" and "you" is very common)
- ✓ Jokes/riddles, teasing and sarcasm can be totally misunderstood
- ✓ Direct attention to context by using a primer word, a hint or cue (make what is not obvious, obvious)
- ✓ State directives in the positive; avoid using "stop" and "don't" – What do you want the student to do rather than what you don't want him to do? ("Walk on the track instead of "Stop walking on the grass." "Walk in the hallway" instead of "Don't run in the hallway.")

<u>Needs Associated with Play</u>

Play is the foundation for a child's cognitive, emotional, language, and social development. But, the obvious question is HOW do we teach play? I think this is an especially hard question as we grow older; face it, as adults, we sometimes forget how to play! Teaching it can be intimidating. There are many terrific resources (listed in Resources) to lead educators in the development of play programming for children with autism. It is beyond the scope of this book to delve into the topic. The following are just some things to consider in a play or early learning program:

- ✓ Teach joint attention and imitation skills first and foremost if not present
- ✓ Teach how to play with toys or imaginary play skills in an isolated setting before having the skills used in a social group (playground)
- ✓ Use picture activity schedules to show the sequence of playing with a toy and more interactive play
- ✓ Use video modelling to demonstrate play sequences (commercial and/or homemade)
- ✓ Use reinforcement to increase play behaviour (remember it is not inherently fun)
- ✓ Use scripts and peers to teach the dialogue and the actions of imaginary play (i.e. set up a pizza counter with a customer, a counter attendant and a cook)

- ✓ Teach play with materials, toys and activities the student enjoys
- ✓ Gradually increase the social interaction of play such as 'dress-up, pretend play (pizza parlour, restaurant) and cooperative games
- ✓ Skills need to be taught and reinforced purposefully - even in social games
- ✓ Rotate the materials used for play to keep kids interested and to expand interest
- ✓ Organize play activities with typically developing peers in order to increase the level of social interaction (Fitness Friends, Recess Buddies, Classwide Social Skills Program™)

Needs Associated with Social and Emotional Understanding

Living with a severe social disorder, deficits in language and sensory challenges must be brutal. Education is incomplete if we fail to address the social and emotional health of a student with autism. Resources that target emotional concerns, affective education and self -regulation are invaluable.

- ✓ Implement systematic programs to directly teach and develop social and emotional understanding (Cognitive Behaviour Therapy, Social Thinking™, The 5 Point Scale, Comic Strip Conversations™)
- ✓ Be sure to make use of teachable moments and natural learning environments to practice and generalize skills learned (never leave learning to isolated skills)
- ✓ Tie emotional and social understanding into the Individual Education Plan so that it is not disregarded
- ✓ Teach students about feelings (give proper names to feelings, identify feelings based on facial expressions, tone of voice and body language, teach physical cues that signal feelings)
- ✓ Teach emotions in context – in real time we never see facial expressions without the context that helps us to understand them

Needs Associated With Dysfunctions in Cognition and Perception

- ✓ Implement visual schedules to identify the steps/activities a child will need to complete; incorporate any changes to the routine and preferred activities; make schedule as interactive as possible (NEVER take it away…it will evolve into a written list)
- ✓ Using graphic organizers helps to reduce the volume of information that must be held in working memory while a student is completing a written or verbal task
- ✓ Focus on a student's understanding of main idea and how new information fits with what is already known (connections will likely not be made without focused teaching)

- ✓ Provide small, clear, step by step instructions (written or pictures or both) when teaching (smaller steps than you might expect are necessary)
- ✓ Develop a tracking system and a reward system to encourage impulse control (staying in seat, reduced interrupting, a token economy that can be exchanged for something that the student values)
- ✓ Play games that provide opportunities to practice categorization
- ✓ Teach student to use visual cues (raising my hand before I speak, waiting for the teacher to call my name, etc...) on desk or in the binder to encourage impulse control
- ✓ Color code binders with specific subjects and classes to facilitate organizing materials (include materials lists that are needed in each subject)
- ✓ Use picture labels and matching to help a student connect activities to places in the room, or materials that they will need
- ✓ Teach new or difficult information using topics of special interest to increase motivation (writing, reading, speaking, math, physical education and so on)
- ✓ Develop rote memory techniques, play recall games (Memory) or develop mnemonic cues (North, East, South, West = Never Eat Shredded Wheat)
- ✓ Explicitly teach students how to use their organizer for homework, assignments and materials (giving them a list is NOT enough)....we must teach its use, provide time in their schedule for it to be used and reinforce its use
- ✓ State in written form (social script) observable behaviours <u>that will be expected</u> in a given social situation (when we are in the assembly we will see you sitting on the chair, hands still, looking at the speaker, etc...). Reprimanding students for what they did wrong after the fact is a waste of time and self esteem
- ✓ Provide opportunities to analyze people's facial expressions, role play and dramatize different states of mind...this teaching needs to be explicit
- ✓ "Debrief" a social situation before it happens - explain what will happen and use social scripts whenever possible (e.g. a fire alarm, a visit to the doctor, a guest speaker visit)
- ✓ Use Carol Grays's Social Stories™ or write simple social scripts to explain social situations (lining up, playing Bingo, greeting an acquaintance, supply teachers)
- ✓ Study and play games with mental state vocabulary: believe, figure, forget, guess, estimate, idea, trick, deceive etc...
- ✓ Use concrete materials to teach abstract concepts (the concept of finished, start, change, time, more, less etc...)
- ✓ Always use examples from the student's own experiences whenever possible - talking through and acting out mental state situations

- ✓ 'Discuss' social situations or problems by creating stick figure drawings of people involved –include thought bubbles to discuss and record what the people might be thinking
- ✓ Provide structure to the thinking task by identifying categories of ideas or a narrower perspective. By narrowing the thinking you are giving the student a starting point or a 'better net.'
- ✓ Ask probing questions to guide thinking: What are ways your mother might use a paper clip? What is something you like to do in the winter? What school subjects might the character in the story like best?
- ✓ Demonstrate often how one can think through the steps and materials needed for a specific experience or activity (going to the pool, a birthday party, a field trip…)
- ✓ Encourage imaginative behaviour by playing "what if" games
- ✓ Teach the student to focus on relevant features within a problem – use a highlighter in text or role play situations to determine what are the important pieces of information
- ✓ Teach exceptions rather than rules (along with the rules)

Needs Associated with Memory

- ✓ Ask "What are you going to do next?" "Tell me what you are going to read." (Then observe to see if student understood the instruction)
- ✓ Reduce working memory loads: Reduce information given to child, break instructions into smaller steps, increase meaningfulness and familiarity of material, simplify language
- ✓ Purposefully point out the relevant details in stories, social situations and explain how the details give us the meaning
- ✓ Visual organizers such as Venn Diagrams, T Charts and Story Boards are excellent tools to introduce and develop concepts
- ✓ Provide plenty of repetition (can be supplied by teacher, learning support or other pupils)
- ✓ Use wall charts, memory cards, visual and audio aides to enhance encoding information in long term memory (Be sure to explicitly teach and practice making the connection! It will not happen otherwise.)
- ✓ Accessorize! Wear hats, masks, or full costumes to enhance the learning experience and explicitly point out the connection between content and accessories
- ✓ Daily journals help to build episodic memory (Have student spend 10-15 minutes writing down what happened to him that day. Where he went, what he did, any interesting things that happened. Be sure to write the day of the week and the date at

the top of each entry. Start the next day by rereading the previous day's entry. Consistent review will help build the memory and teach student to attend to things worth remembering.)

Needs Associated with Shifting Attention and Other Executive Functions

Executive function skills require individualized, structured and direct teaching in real life contexts. It is not enough to provide the tools such as an agenda book, an organizer or checklist and hope the student will follow through. Intensive practice with immediate feedback is essential. Just as important is the gradual withdrawl of adult prompting (fading) so that the skill may become more of an automatic habit. Executive function goals should really be linked to every academic subject because they are an intricate aspect of a student's ability to act on what he or she knows.

- ✓ Ensure that you have the student's attention before you begin to give instructions (Eye contact may interfere with listening....it may be wise not to ask for it)
- ✓ Implement a visual schedule that identifies the steps/activities that a child will need to complete; incorporate any changes to the routine and preferred activities (NEVER take it away)
- ✓ Minimize and preview changes in the routine and transitions
- ✓ Use a transition object or card that is embedded into the daily schedule and routine so that a student knows when the activity is finished and it is time to change activities (putting the basketball away indicates the end of gym)
- ✓ Use distracting toys, sensory tools or a hand clap to signify a change (we use a shiny "disco ball" which helps to shift attention from one person or task to another)
- ✓ A "First – Then" visual board helps the student to know what he must do first in order to shift to the next event
- ✓ Indicate how long student would work on a specific question or assignment (use a Time Timer™ to indicate the time visually)
- ✓ Write the change on a whiteboard or blank paper without verbal communication
- ✓ Use of timers or buzzers to signal the end of one activity and the beginning of the next (some students will be agitated by these)
- ✓ Given training in a self-regulatory routine, such as Goal, Plan, Do, Check visual cues and fading prompts, student will (verbally or nonverbally) identify tasks that are easy or difficult for him, explain why and request help when tasks are difficult (Kenworthy et. al, 2014).

Needs Associated with Auditory Processing Difficulty

- ✓ Use visual organizers, labels, instructions, steps, schedules, concrete objects and every kind of visual input to give information

- ✓ Teach nonverbal communication skills (body language, gestures, tone of voice) so that the student is more likely to "read" non- verbal behaviour even if they have difficulty processing what someone has said
- ✓ Pair visuals (pictures and objects) with auditory information so that the student eventually attaches meaning to the auditory input
- ✓ Plan activities around discriminating sounds (sounds in the environment, shaking sounds, letter sounds, sound patterns etc…)
- ✓ Provide plenty of processing time
- ✓ Use visual cues for instructions, steps, starting tasks, ending tasks etc…
- ✓ Keep verbal instruction to a minimum: state the bottom line – short and simple
- ✓ Provide extra "wait time" after verbal instructions are given (once you repeat the question you are starting the processing time over!)
- ✓ Teach self -advocacy skills so that a student is able to express a need for processing time, visual supports and cues ("Give me a minute, I'm thinking.")

Needs Associated with Sensory Regulation

When negative behaviour arises it is wise to first look at sensory issues that may be upsetting a child. Remember that even students with high functioning autism cannot always express what is bothering them. Sensory regulation issues are especially critical for those students who have no way of expressing their discomfort or needs.

- ✓ Teach student how to request a break verbally, in written form, using objects or cue cards
- ✓ Teach the student how to communicate sensory needs by teaching the use of picture symbols of various sensory concerns (lights, heat, cold, loud, various sense organs such as the ears, mouth, nose and eyes) so that the child has a way to "locate" and express the problem
- ✓ Dim the lights, use an incandescent lamp, change the fluorescent lighting
- ✓ Place tennis balls on the bottom of chair legs to ease the "scratchy noise"
- ✓ Mute the P. A system in a classroom
- ✓ Provide a listening center where students can "regroup" with preferred music
- ✓ Provide earplugs or headphones/music while student is working
- ✓ Prepare a quiet area for break - use a small decorative water/Zen fountain (this works wonders!) or a white noise machine if the student likes it
- ✓ Create sensory bins with items of various smells and textures and incorporate sensory time into the student's daily schedule

- ✓ Make use of the tools that are prescribed by Occupational Therapists; having items packed away in a box is counterproductive

<u>Needs Associated with Behavioural Issues</u>

What need does a student's behaviour communicate? When a newborn infant cries her parents learn to detect differences in the cries. Parents can interpret what the baby wants by the cry the child expresses. Although autistic people are not babies, they have difficulty by nature, in expressing their needs. This is true for both verbal and non-verbal persons. It is especially acute when the individual is under stress of some kind. We must never set out to change behaviour without first learning what the behaviour is telling us. How?

- ✓ Keep logs of behaviours and their context- when do they happen? What is the child doing when the behaviour occurs? What are other people doing when it occurs? What in the environment or the situation could he be trying to tell us about? This is an informal behaviour assessment where we look to see patterns in behaviour and responses to behaviour.

- ✓ Invite a behaviour resource person into the class to conduct a Functional Behaviour Assessment or do one yourself

Possible ways to facilitate the problem solving process:

<u>Positive Behaviour Support Plans</u>

1. Identify the problem behaviour occurring : be VERY specific about what is observed, not what is assumed (someone should be able to perform the behaviour based on your objective description)

2. Identify the function of the behaviour and contributing factors (attention, tangible, escape, avoidance): What is the child trying to tell you? What autistic thinking might be triggering this behaviour?

3. Identify a more appropriate alternative behaviour: preferably an action that will replace the less desired action.

4. Develop strategies for replacing the inappropriate behaviour with the alternative behaviour. Shape replacement behaviours that are more appropriate. Reinforce a behaviour that is more acceptable and that can be performed instead of an inappropriate behaviour. Replacement behaviour makes the unwanted behaviour ineffective or irrelevant because it no longer serves the function as well as the replacement behaviour.

   For example, if the student is constantly biting his fingers, introduce a squeeze ball or vibrating ball and use prompts and reinforcement to "shape" the use of the ball instead of the biting.

5. Develop the behaviour intervention plan. Ensure that it is followed by EVERYONE (classroom staff, administration, custodial staff and any volunteers).

6. Evaluate the behaviour intervention plan: Was the behaviour reduced? Was a more positive or appropriate behaviour increased? **Were the child's needs met?**

It is imperative that all people who work with the student are familiar with the plan. Consistency is critical for internalization and generalization of appropriate behaviour.

<u>Present new stimuli</u>
Something new can help to get a student "unstuck." Try to avoid talking the student out of his anxiety (it doesn't work). Instead, stay quiet and start playing with a puzzle or another object that interests the child. Squeeze a sensory tool. Sometimes it is enough just to be near the student pretending to be working on a puzzle or reading a favourite book. Doing so can create a distraction and offer a way out of a one track mind.

<u>Routines</u>
Familiar routines bring about a sense of calm and reassurance for students with autism. This is much like the way that babies and small children are soothed into sleep when they have a regular bedtime routine. Implement routines for clean-up times, putting books away, study sessions, silent reading, transition times and so on. (This is a great tool for all students).

<u>Sensory stimulation</u>
Offering a sensory room or physical exercise before classes begin can offset anxiety building up between home and school. Physical exercise is widely underestimated as a way to release stress, build positive emotions and clear thinking. Students with autism need to have regular exercise breaks throughout their day and yet, so often they do not.

<u>Maintain your own composure</u>
The only thing worse than a student who is having a meltdown is a student **and** a teacher having meltdowns! Maintain the student's dignity at all times. The way a teacher handles an emotional meltdown models for all students how to treat a person with autism. Allowing ourselves to lose control, taking behaviour personally or being offended by a child's behaviour is, in my opinion, selfish. A student who cannot cope with a sensory and cognitive system that is very different from our own is not to be belittled or antagonized under any circumstances. It is never right. We would never accept that for our own children or those we love.

Needs Associated with Leisure

Sadly, too often children with autism grow into adults that do not know what to do with their free time. Free time can be extremely stressful or just a waste of time and talents for some individuals with autism. A child engaged in an activity provide parents with some desperately needed time for themselves – even if it is to go to the washroom!

The development of play and leisure skills begins in the early years of schooling is an important component of education planning in every year of school. In adulthood, work placements take minimal time and down time is often abundant. Many adults with autism simply don't have a range of interests nor the skills needed to develop connections within the community.

Consider how individual interests might be used to help a student develop connections outside of the classroom. The online world has certainly been able to reduce isolation and bring together people who have less typical interests: Yu-Gi-Oh! Or The Gathering® clubs, science fiction clubs, computer/technology clubs, chess clubs, military history clubs and so on offer a world beyond work or school. The goal is to develop activities in which the individual can independently engage and enjoy the time spent. Keep the following ideas in mind when planning the teaching of independent leisure skills:

- ✓ Leisure and play skills are personal and should be based on the individual's interests (not on the interests of parents or teachers or what we might think the individual *should* enjoy)
- ✓ Ensure that the student is able to perform the leisure activity independently after it has been taught and generalized (work yourself out of a job)
- ✓ Involve the student in community activities with structure and support (visual and human support)
- ✓ Teach the social skills that go with more social leisure activities (waiting, proximity to people, sharing, cooperation, turn taking, following rules and reciprocity)
- ✓ Be patient: many activities are not enjoyed at first; many need time, routine and structure until the activity becomes familiar, safe and enjoyable
- ✓ Quality of life **is** a real and relevant part of the autism curriculum for individuals with autism

Consider teaching or introducing the students to a variety of experiences throughout the school years:

- Sports (e.g., bowling, swimming, golf, bocce ball,)
- Jogging or long distance running
- Weight lifting
- Arts activities (e.g., music, theatre, movies, sewing, knitting, needlepoint, crafts)
- Nature activities (e.g., camping, hiking, gardening, landscape design)
- Participating in organized groups (e.g., Scouts, chess club, Lego club)
- Attending social events (e.g., dances, religious services, birthday parties, dinner parties, weddings, funerals)
- Using a television, stereo, digital devices, the telephone, phone book
- Pet care
- Playing card games, board games and video games
- Teach online safety
- Visiting art galleries and museums

Needs Associated with Independence

The last aspect of teaching that is the foundation to all other areas of programming is the need to build independence and autonomy for each student with autism. To educate a child is to inherently prepare them for an adult life that is as self -sufficient and autonomous. Life at a school has a way of sucking us into the vortex of tiny details and busyness, blinding us to the larger vision of nurturing the growth and self -actualization of human beings. We can easily lose sight of the big picture.

- ✓ Embedded in our planning must be goals for making every skills increasingly independent (fading prompts)
- ✓ Avoid jumping in to rescue a student - struggle is not bad for a child (if we build in visual supports, prompts and small steps so that a measure of success can be experienced)
- ✓ Gradually increase your physical distance from the student as the student's skills emerge - When teaching a typical child to ride a bike we often hold onto the bicycle and help the child to stabilize the bike. We don't just push the child and hope for the best - we gradually release our grip on the bike and we back away as the child becomes steadier.
- ✓ Incorporate daily activities that the student can do completely free from adult help
- ✓ To the extent possible the environment should be organized so students can do things for themselves: hooks that can reached, utensils and materials that can be accessed and visual supports that outline the steps of a process
- ✓ The more opportunities we give children to do things for themselves the more we allow their esteem to grow - Before you begin to zip up that jacket or install the ink cartridge, ask yourself: with the right support, could the student could do this himself?

Not all individuals will achieve a completely independent lifestyle but it is incumbent upon educators to build autonomy for <u>each and every</u> child. Teaching the skills needed and providing the technology needed so that individuals can make their personal needs, desires and choices known is of paramount importance. When individuals are able to do things for themselves and make decisions regarding their lives, they internalize a sense autonomy and self -confidence. Plus, a sense of empowerment goes a long way to reduce anxiety and behaviour issues.

Building the Foundation of an Authentic IEP

What is this Crazy Little Thing Called an IEP?

All patients benefit from differentiated health care. What is a reasonable treatment for one may be deadly for another. All students benefit from differentiated instruction. Each human is created with differences in abilities and ways of learning. Even within a family, each child has his or her own temperament, personality and chronological order which in turn impacts the way we parent each child individually. One child's emotional, physical, intellectual needs are quite different from another within the same home! It's no wonder that in many ways, all students require an 'individual education plan.'

This is particularly true of students that have an Autism Spectrum Disorder because each of these students present the education system with a complex myriad of skills, strengths, deficits and learning styles that demand a differentiated approach to programming. If we don't individualize programming, resources and assessment, I fear that we end up 'warehousing' a student rather than authentically educating a student.

An Individual Education Plan or a plan by another name is a definite record of a plan of action for the educational program of a student. It is a roadmap that states where a student *is* currently, and where the student *is going* as a 'whole' individual. By whole, I mean academically AND emotionally, behaviourally, physically, socially and cognitively. An effective IEP is a culmination of collaborative sharing of insights, goals, objectives and resources (both human and material).

An IEP is also a government mandated legal document for students with special needs. The special needs of students are not left to chance or to the good will of teachers. Our laws protect them.

What's the Point of an IEP? Does it Really Matter?

Imagine for a moment that you finally have the means to build your 'dream home.' This will be the culmination of your hard work, dreams and sacrifices. You have painstakingly chosen the right contractor and the perfect location. You have worked closely with an architect to ensure that every detail is well thought out. Now, imagine that the contractor began digging the foundation and building the beloved structure before consulting the floor plan and blueprints!

Blueprints, floor plans, and consultation bring structure and common vision to building a dream home. The homeowners need to have their ideas and input valued and the builder needs to have a plan that is detailed enough to keep him "on track" and within budget.

The same could be said for teachers, professionals and parents of individuals with autism. Each has a perspective that is valuable in forming a plan for the education of the student. Each person who knows the child's needs and strengths holds a 'piece' of the full image of the child. Each piece of the whole child image corresponds to developmental goals that must be acknowledged. Goals are just wishes if they aren't written and accompanied by a plan of action.

Still not convinced? Imagine being in the hospital undergoing extensive testing to determine the cause of a debilitating illness. Based on the symptoms reported, medical staff call for tests to be done. Results of those tests determine the course of treatment. Patients rely on the fact that doctors and nurses follow a plan; they use the results of tests to provide information as to the course of treatment. There is **not** a lot of tolerance in the medical field for trial and error, guesswork and lack of knowledge!

Our health depends on the calculated implementation of an action plan. So too does the construction of a building. As parents and educators we have been given the privilege of nurturing a child and guiding him to his full potential. We can never take this privilege for granted. We must never leave a child's development to chance or good intentions. Consider how successful a diet or exercise plan is if it is left to good intentions. Each and every student with autism deserves to have a team of people that have a genuine and selfless interest in promoting that student's educational goals. Educators are a critical part of the village that cultivates a child to become the individuals they were created to be.

The importance of the document cannot be overstated. Without a definitive plan we are just well intentioned builders, making decisions as we go and hoping for a dream result. An IEP is useful when it:

- ☑ Records realistic and meaningful goals
- ☑ Determines the degree of support needed for learning
- ☑ Provides coherent, specific plans for focusing learning activities
- ☑ Is reviewed frequently to determine progress towards goals
- ☑ Facilitates communication and provides accountability
- ☑ Documents the use of adaptive/assistive technologies
- ☑ Shared openly with all team members

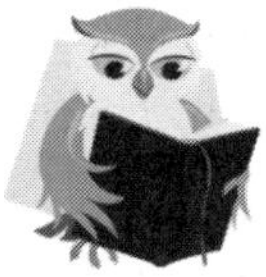

The teacher who does not understand that it is necessary to teach autistic children seemingly obvious things will feel impatient and irritated.

Hans Asperger

What *IS* an Authentic IEP and What is it *NOT*?

An Authentic IEP is NOT:

☒ A comprehensive script covering the details of daily programming

☒ A plan for only the most severely disabled students

☒ A product developed by one educator planning in isolation

☒ A plan that is restricted to changes made to academic curriculum

☒ Limited to the resources available in the classroom or school

☒ A pristine document that should be protected from overuse

☒ A formal "hoop" that all educators must jump through in order to meet the expectations of their school board and their government

☒ A generic plan that is impersonal; a "one size fits all" sort of document

An Authentic IEP IS:

☑ A realistic and manageable written plan of action for a student who requires accommodations or modifications to the regular school program in order to access the curriculum and experience growth

☑ A plan to address the student's autism needs through the alternative expectations (outside state or provincial curriculum such as sensory issues, behaviour goals, social communication and language skills)

☑ A flexible, working document that begs to be revised according to the student's progress towards specified goals

☑ A plan that matches the student's priority needs and strengths to teaching strategies, learning opportunities and assessment practices

☑ A legal document that educators are responsible to create within a month of the start of school and use daily

☑ A summary of the student's strengths and needs (skills), goals and performance objectives and timelines towards meeting these objectives

☑ A plan incorporating the programming decisions of other service providers (Speech and Language pathology, Occupational Therapy, etc.) and linking them to the daily instruction the student receives

☑ The product of a collaborative effort of key persons involved with the child which is deliberately shared and open to persons directly involved with the child's education (paraprofessionals, parents, administrators)

If an IEP is so Important, What is the Problem?

A Little Perspective Goes a Long Way

Given an emphasis on the essential nature of collaboration in the education of a student with autism, it seems fair and hopefully helpful to provide some perspective from the people who love and care for these individuals. Real collaboration depends on a genuine understanding of the different perspectives of the people who love this child.

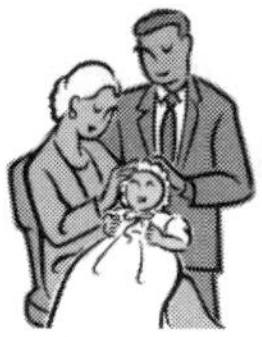

A Parent's Point of View...

When the diagnosis of autism was given to our only son, our world fell apart in a way that no words could ever describe. Without consciously knowing it we had built a set of expectations around raising a boy and all that goes with his development into a man. We had dreams of sporting events, hordes of teenage males eating us out of house and home, girlfriends, parties, college and eventually marriage and grandchildren. With an autism diagnosis every one of those dreams seemed shattered. Words like "severe social and communication impairments, restricted repetitive and stereotyped patterns of behaviour, interests, and activities, and lack of symbolic or imaginative play," became the catch words for describing our son - and his future. Kieran was positioned on the far left of the autism spectrum: severe, classic autism. Our lives had changed forever.

A diagnosis brought with it, guilt, grief, denial and anger. To be fair, it even brought some comfort. At least now we finally had a name for what was wrong. But a diagnosis also marked the beginning of an upward climb that at times seemed more than we could take. Well- meaning family and friends questioned the diagnosis. They tried to reassure us that their children "did that too!" Well educated family members discounted the diagnosis of autism. Our son was, after all, "very social and active." Thus, in the minds of some, he could not possibly have autism. In spite of three separate diagnoses by different doctors over a few years we found ourselves trying to debate or convince disbelievers, including family.

Our circle of friends diminished as our little boy's needs made it almost impossible to enjoy anything social. We threw ourselves into researching therapies and learning how to parent our child. Time seemed to slow down at a time when we needed it to speed up. Waiting lists were excruciating as we watched our little boy slip away from us. We felt isolated, helpless and lost.

I have had the privilege of meeting many, many families that tell me that our story mirrors their experiences. From the moment of birth, children with autism demand more of their parents' time, energy, marriage and finances than typical children. In addition, an autism diagnosis for one child changes the lives of siblings. In all honesty, no one in the family is unaffected. Not even the family dog.

Waiting lists, assessments, therapies, meltdowns and dietary difficulties make living a "normal life" quite complicated! Just coordinating appointments for specialists, and therapists, tutors and group activities is mind boggling! This, in addition to the fact that our children with autism don't cope well without structure and routine! Parents become overwhelmed, weary and sometimes cynical because from the moment they know something isn't quite right with their child they dive into a world where the same questions are asked time and again. The heart wrenching story of your child's developmental difficulties needs to be retold and relived over and over again with each new professional and situation. Autism doesn't sleep or take a holiday. At times, challenges seem insurmountable as emotional and physical strength wane while parents try to find their way through innumerable obstacles. Times of change, bedtimes, mealtimes and daily errands become too much to bear. Family outings can be a source of stress and discord. Many marriages don't survive; a child's needs engulf a family and tear some apart.

I share our story, not to garner sympathy, but rather, to help the reader gain awareness - awareness of a lifestyle that is in many ways indescribable. These are the scars that parents bring with them to school every year. Some parents may be reluctant and apprehensive about sending their child to school, for fear the staff may misunderstand him or not know how to cope with his behaviour and learning needs. Many of our children can't tell us about their day; it may only be reflected in their behaviour. Even when a student *seems* to be very articulate, most parents will have NO clue as to what he is doing and how he is coping during the six hours that he is away from us.

Parents of autistic children begin their parenting career agonizing over what *feels* wrong with our child, having to wait for a proper diagnosis and then fight to get a child from waiting lists to therapy. Parents spend an inordinate amount of time advocating for various services and assessments and unconsciously, building resentment towards a system that, by and large, has few answers and even fewer resources. We tend to over spend our physical and emotional energy trying to get our child the support he or she needs so badly. At the same time, we grope through the dark trying to learn how to parent children who are neurologically wired differently. Most likely, the way we were raised will **not** work for our kids with autism. Add to the angst, the judgmental stares and disturbing comments delivered by those who believe they have the monopoly on the 'correct' methods of parenting.

Parents spend an inordinate amount of time advocating for various services and assessments and unconsciously, building resentment towards a system that, by and large, has few answers and even fewer resources.

Without consciously meaning to, parents tend to bring the internalized "fight or flight" approach to their child's school experience. Unfortunately, it is ingrained in many. Some may have an underlying mistrust of the school system based on real experiences or the media. But, I think it's safe to say that most parents really just want someone to care about and value their child. We need someone to walk with us, affirm us as parents and to help us to educate and celebrate our child. We want to collaborate, not dictate. We need the school to welcome and love our child just the way he is – unconditionally.

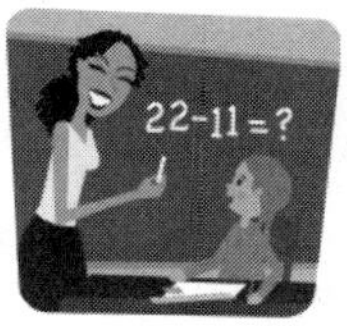

A Teacher's Point of View...

I believe that the majority of teachers enter the profession with a strong desire to 'reach' children: a burning aspiration to nurture the cognitive, physical, emotional, social and spiritual growth of a child. Some may accuse me of being idealistic, but I maintain that, after 20 plus years of teaching experience, the majority of educators have the child's best interest at heart. Our intentions are good and noble.

The burning desire to cultivate minds soon meets with the reality of nurturing dozens of students. A teacher has the arduous task of meeting the needs of each and every student for whom he or she has responsibility every day, all day. I can personally attest to the fact that differentiating the curriculum and teaching methods is no simple feat. Neither is finding time to listen to each story and every heartache. It is absolutely necessary, but challenging, even for the most seasoned professionals. Add the need for effective classroom management and efficient use of human and material resources and the task becomes a really tough one.

Teaching a classroom of students is a balancing act like no other. Think of how difficult it can be to meet each child's needs in a single family and then multiply that by at least twenty! Have you have ever struggled with guilt because you failed to spend quality time with each of your children in a day or to give them the attention they needed? Imagine how that must feel for a teacher who needs to carve time, attention and patience for 20 or more students. Each child comes with their own distinct personality, interests, weaknesses and abilities. Each arrives with stories that need to be told and needs that scream to be met.

Any parent or adult who has hosted a birthday party for a child has had a taste of what it is like to care for and attend to the needs of more than a family of children. Entertaining all of the stories, questions and concerns of party guests for a couple of hours is enough to induce a coma like sleep. Teachers have the responsibility of being the entertainment director plus educating each of these children each and every day. It really helps build relationship when parents appreciate and empathize with this fact of classroom life.

The excitement of the start of the school year soon turns from honeymoon to a roller coaster that one cannot stop. The reality is that there is no time to lose. Those precious days in the first month need to be spent getting to know each child, pouring over assessments, reports, students' histories and talking to parents. But, there are 20 or more children and deadlines for Individual Education Plans must be met. Fear that somehow we do not have what it takes to teach such a complex child, doubt in our own abilities and a lack of professional development and resources weigh heavily on the mind of a teacher.

Teachers feel the pressure of providing time for each child daily, meeting government curriculum expectations and communicating with parents. This is to take place while we assess student learning, evaluate our own teaching and carry on with the housekeeping and extracurricular aspects of school life. Yes, teaching is exhausting emotionally and physically! As I write this I cannot help but feel sorry for our own family members who live with us!

To be completely frank, teaching a student with autism often sparks a sense of trepidation in educators. Negative media and horror stories of litigious conflicts leave many teachers feeling ill prepared to meet the challenge. Autism presents a daunting and intimidating task for even experienced autism specialists. No one autistic child is like another and many teachers are fearful of failing the student with autism.

Educators want the child to learn and grow. We want the best for the child. We want parents to know that we do care and that we will do our best with what we have. We want to collaborate and share the experience. We need to be supported and affirmed when possible. We need to learn from each other and with each other.

Losing Perspective

The new school year roars in with the promise of a fresh start and the race to get IEPs completed is on. Legal obligations keep us accountable but I fear that many times the products produced are just that – products. In spite of good intentions, many barriers keep IEPS from being authentic and useful!

Too many times, Special Education teachers are left to create and distribute the plan to the teachers who will be delivering it! Classroom teachers who haven't played a part in preparing it will be less likely to 'buy into it' with the level of commitment that is necessary. Some teachers think that the IEP is a "special education" entity unto itself and they may miss the relevance it has to their day to-day teaching and assessment.

Having one or two teachers stay late after school to create a document that winds up in an official student record or in a filing cabinet can be a waste of time as well. A pristine document that is technically 'done,' but, won't see the light of day until report card time rolls around, is hardly useful. To make matters worse, the document may only come out of the drawer if someone knows that it needs to be reviewed! If not, it remains hidden and useless.

The dreaded reprint is another IEP horror! Amid the urgency of deadlines and the self-doubt of a well- intentioned teacher, generic copies of previous years' educational plans make their way into a parent's hands. Big mistake. Many plans consist of outdated and obsolete goals that need to be shredded! I assure you that nothing is more disheartening for a parent, than to witness the reincarnation of their child's goals in the exact same form every year! Experiencing the "never changing IEP" feels like having someone say to your face: "Your child is just not making any progress. There is no hope; no way. Your child cannot grow." Ouch.

With the best of intentions we ask the student's parents to be involved in planning but they sense (real or otherwise) that their role is merely a token of collaboration. We know that parental input *can* be viewed superficially. In that case, asking for input is a waste of time. Let's be real. If we ask for a parent's knowledge of their child and goals for the child's future, the least we can do is to genuinely listen to what they have to say, and then, do what we can to incorporate their contribution.

Educators can sometimes stand in judgment of parents who fail to participate in their child's education. I admit it, I have been guilty of this more than I care to remember. I have to remind myself that in spite of a deep love for their child, parents can be so depleted from the task of raising their child with autism that they can't muster the energy to join the work of educating their child. Many parents just need someone else to take on a part of their responsibility so they leave education up to the school. Judging another is far easier than recognizing a need and taking action to offer support. At the same time, experience has taught me that we can only change what is in our control. The Serenity Prayer often comes to mind when I am challenged to "find the courage to change the things I am able to change and to accept the things I cannot change." If a parent cannot be involved, I must do what I can with what I have.

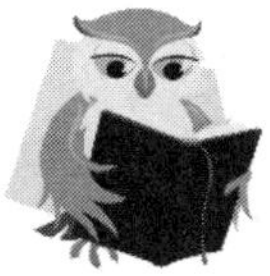

"Do what you can, with what you have, where you are."

Theodore Roosevelt

"I am going to be your worst nightmare this year! Don't even think of making a wrong move!" Yes, some parents do say that! They come into a new school year with an offensive stance towards staff. Not surprisingly, this approach only serves to put a wedge into the relationship with the people who will care for and educate their child for six hours of the day! Do you feel inspired to be your best for someone who threatens you? Maybe for the short term. But, it is human nature to be motivated and inspired to be our best when we are affirmed and valued. Threats and intimidation may win the battle but rest assured, those who use them, will lose the war.

Last but not least, parents have shared that their biggest complaint with IEPs is that they fail to link meaningfully to the day to day activities and subjects of their children. The IEP team needs to be sure that what is written in the plan IS translated into an actual action in the classroom. Many "autism" goals can be weaved into the regular curriculum. Social skills, executive function, self- regulation can be written into the IEP, embedded within the daily activities and monitored daily. When the plan is developed by more than one person, with a sound understanding of the student's learning strengths and needs and realistic, relevant goals are set, the IEP stands a chance of being useful.

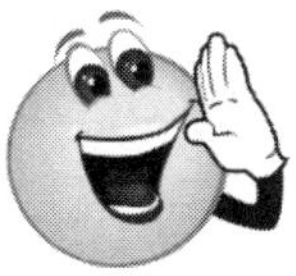

An effective educational plan is authentic, child centered, practical, measurable, meaningful and utilized regularly!

Breaking Down the Barriers: No Teacher or Parent is an Island

Even though it is not always mandated by some higher power called 'government' or 'administration,' the most effective way to ensure that an IEP reflects the 'whole student' is to create opportunities for collaboration. At times, this word sends shivers down the spine of educators and parents alike because it requires them to discuss, share, listen and compromise. No, this is NOT an easy task.

"It takes a village to raise a child." This could not be truer than in the education of a child with special needs, such as autism. When we invite parents, teachers, special education teachers, principals, speech and language pathologists, occupational therapists, psychologists, behaviour specialists, outside agencies and even the student (when possible) to provide their unique perspective we are building a more authentic plan for a student. Yes, I know it sounds overwhelming. But, the observations, information and vision of key persons involved in a child's education are invaluable because each and every person sees the child from a different perspective. Together these perspectives help to provide a more comprehensive and real picture of the individual. A student is not the sum of his or her academic and cognitive strengths and weaknesses. Rather, a student is a whole person with physical, emotional, social, intellectual and spiritual facets that must be recognized, nurtured and developed. The key here is to invite people who know the child – knowing beyond assessment data.

Being in a classroom alone with 25 students or more can sometimes feel very lonely. Any single parent can probably relate to the overwhelming feeling of bearing the responsibility of raising children on one set of shoulders. It's pretty normal for teachers to feel isolated, ill-equipped and overwhelmed. Just as it is important for parents to reach out for help, so too, should teachers. Seeking the knowledge of colleagues that are positive and affirming is essential to being the best you can be for your students. Nurturing relationships with other professionals such as speech and language pathologists, occupational therapists, special education teachers and community agencies builds a teacher's ability to widen his or her knowledge base and strategy toolbox. We can offer a student more if we open ourselves up to the various perspectives and expertise of others. I cannot help but think that like no other students, those with autism force us to move beyond our islands and reach out for others.

> ***We can offer a student more if we open ourselves up to the various perspectives and expertise of others.***

Meetings are a waste of time, unless people come to a meeting prepared to share their insight and the opportunity is given for sharing. Parents should have equal opportunity to share their insights, ask for clarification and pose questions. I highly recommend that parents and teachers take the time, before a meeting, to consider their own visions or priorities with regards to the child's education. By recording thoughts prior to meeting, we will surely feel more valuable to the team. It can be intimidating for parents to sit amongst a group of professionals. Teachers can feel equally intimidated. By having a record in front of you, it is more likely that you'll be able to maintain your train of thought and contribute constructively to the conversation. Appendix A entitled, Portrait of a Student, is a template, which could be used for the purpose of recording pertinent information informally before a school meeting. This guide provides questions that keep the discussion meaningful and on track. It is very challenging to pull ideas out of your head when you have the attention of many sets of eyes.

Whether we are parents or educators, we probably all know how brutal it can be to keep an open ear and mind while listening to another person. We tend to listen on a surface level while we quietly construct our response or defense. Looking back at some of the most emotionally charged meetings with parents, I have learned that even the most 'difficult' parents are just saying: "I love my child deeply and I want the absolute best there is for him." In the same way, a teacher is often saying: "I want to do my very best for your child. I can only do what I know with the resources that are available. Please do not assume that I am acting with malice."

As a parent of a child with autism the best meetings I have participated in were those in which we all left our 'gloves' at the door, focused on growth and positive facts first. Highlighting the positive made a softer forum for dealing with the hard stuff. There were many times that I had to put my political advocate role 'on hold' so that I could really listen and hear what the educational team was saying. It's not that I compromised my son's education. It was more a matter of choosing my battles and knowing that if I expected to be respected and valued, and if I wanted my voice to be heard, then I needed to extend the same courtesy. Threats of legal action, rallying the troops and going above someone's head may win a battle but rarely do these actions result in winning the war. The long term cost to parent and student is extraordinary. Rather than compromise my son's educational program, I think that a collegial, compromising and optimistic attitude served him far better.

The various educational teams with whom I have collaborated regarding my own child's needs have worked with integrity to provide the best services, resources and programs that they could offer. This is not to say that there were no differences in opinion. There were plenty! Many times I knew the school team was as frustrated with me, as I was with them. It was just a matter of not allowing resentment, accusations and blame to enter into the discussion. I believe that that is a choice we each make. The fact is that, although I am there to advocate for my child's needs, the educators too, must advocate for all of the students' needs. The needs of one cannot override the needs of many.

As a teacher, the most effective meetings that I have been a part of were the meetings where every member was made to feel welcomed and valued. Allowing parents to voice their thoughts, opinions and concerns without any interruption (unless there is a personal verbal attack on an individual) provides them a chance to vent their thoughts and anxiety. Remember, parents often come to meetings intimidated, defensive and fearful of being ambushed. They may come across as being pushy or on the offensive but that is more often than not a matter of nervous energy or anxiety. As a teacher, I feel that it is my responsibility to listen with an open heart and mind to the essence of the message and not the tone of the voice. I have to keep in mind that parents of autistic children usually have keen observations of their children and many do know a great deal about autism. It is up to me to check my ego and listen. For the parents who are less capable of expressing their thoughts, I feel it is equally important for me to get off of my academic pedestal and guide them through the process - always being mindful that I have been granted a privilege to touch their child's life.

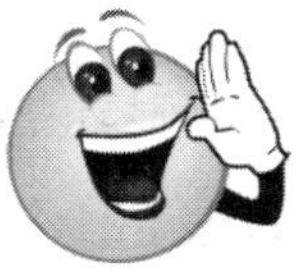

Optimism Fuels Collaboration

Optimism is a way of looking at life and its inherent stresses. Does the concept of an optimistic person conjure an image of an overly joyful, seemingly naïve and perky individual in your mind? I would challenge that notion. True optimists choose to look for opportunity in the middle of adversity. They allow themselves and others to feel emotion – even raw, unruly emotion. Optimists are open to the venting of feelings but they summon an inner structure that reframes their thoughts back to a belief that adversity is temporary. Hardships can be overcome by a 'can do' attitude perseverance and a powerful belief that all will work for the good.

An educational meeting regarding the life of a child is naturally an emotionally charged environment. I would argue that the need for optimism is paramount. In my experience optimism is the only lens through which to view planning an education for an individual with autism. It is through this lens that we recognize and celebrate opportunities for growth. To invite doubt, resentment and negativity to a meeting for a child is counter-productive. These attitudes only breed defensiveness and pessimism which, in effect, stains the way that we approach a student with autism.

Most importantly, "children learn what they live," and as the adults in a child's life, is it not our responsibility to model a "growth mindset" and an attitude of positive persistence and hope? When we think and act as if a child will be successful, we enable the child to think positively about their own challenges. Our students deserve an optimistic team in which every member is determined to develop the child's potential and make the team work!

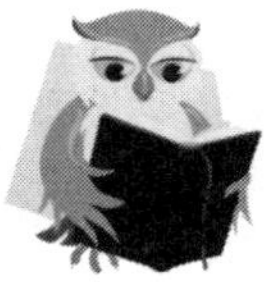

A positive thinker does not refuse to recognize the negative; he refuses to dwell on it. Positive thinking is a form of thought which habitually looks for the best results from the worst conditions.

Norman Vincent Peale

When Teams Don't Work the Way They Should

Okay, I am the first one to admit that there are those folks who just don't want to play nice. For one reason or another, and there can be multitudes of reasons, we will meet those who cannot get past some deep drive that limits their effectiveness in working as a team. The collaboration of many minds is the goal, but the game doesn't stop if someone refuses to play! We must work with what we've got. To put it metaphorically: we have to 'bloom where we are planted.'

At times like these we rely on those wise words, once again: "Lord, help me to accept the things I cannot change, courage to change the things I can; and the wisdom to know the difference." Sometimes we have to put our 'big girl pants' (or big boy) and silently ask for a double dose of optimism, open mindedness and creativity. The bottom line is that the child is the center of the process. We've always got to meet the needs of the child so we have to build an educational plan with the ideas, the professional and parental perspectives and the resources that we <u>do</u> have. Dwelling on what we don't have is counterproductive. The child is not as well represented without the effort and input of a whole team, but the child's <u>needs</u> remain the same and as professionals we cannot forsake giving the best we've got to that child.

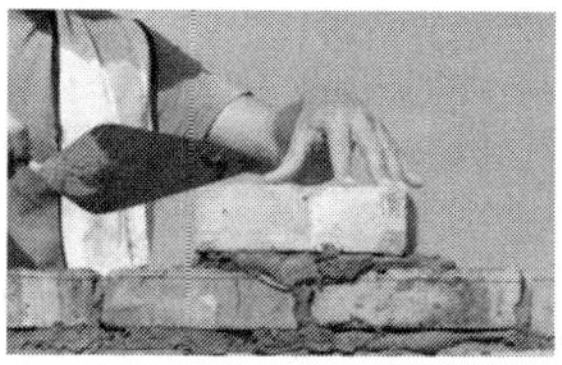

Where do we Start?

When should IEP meetings occur? How often?

Keep in mind that in the United States it is mandatory to hold a formal IEP meeting at least once a year. If we are not mandated to host a formal IEP meeting, the adage, "the sooner the better" is an appropriate response to the question of when IEP meetings should occur. I have to admit that I cringe when I hear about some long, drawn out and tortuous IEP meetings! I cannot help but think that this is a nasty way to 'build relationship' and develop trust between parents and educators. It also seems to obstruct the road to consistent communication between teachers and parents because it would appear to 'suck the life' out of that relationship!

While arduous meetings may be out of our control, we do maintain the power to decide how we will approach our relationship with parents. The more we are able to invite regular and brief communication with a student's parent, the less chance there will be of a communication breakdown. Because the start of the year is so crazy and I am not in a jurisdiction that mandates IEP meetings, I send home the "Portrait of a Student" template. The ideas sent to me by the parents on this template as well as documentation found in the student records help us to begin to get a sense of direction in planning and to create the first draft of the IEP.

Keeping parents aware of and involved in educational issues, concerns or program changes is imperative because they have a right to know what involves their child. When time permits a formal or informal meeting is organized with the parents and personnel that are involved with the student. A list of possible participants is included below. Contacting parents through an informal or formal note, a phone call and/or an email to let them know when discussions with a team member have led to changes in the IEP is crucial. This is formally done at report card time but would be appreciated at any time. Communication builds trust and a solid foundation for a collegial relationship.

Who Should be Involved?

The IEP meeting or any formal meeting regarding the student's educational plan, should include the following:

Parents – Purposely placed at the top of the list. Parents are a valuable resource when we are trying to get to know a child. Parents witness the day to day behaviour, sensory issues, skills, interests, fears and problems that a child with ASD exhibits. Parents have key information on how the child responds to 'real life' in grocery stores, restaurants, and other public places. They can provide critical information that will help to prioritize goals and objectives.

At least one **Classroom Teacher** -Teachers are able to provide firsthand accounts and observations of daily life in the classroom (which can vary significantly from home life). They should bring to the meeting their observations based on reports, assessments, anecdotal notes, and data collection. Avoid bringing subjective value laden judgments such as: "John is a manipulative child who always disrupts the class." (Do you really think you will inspire support and willingness to compromise when you speak like that?)

At least one **Special Education Teacher** – Special Education Teachers will have the specialized knowledge of Autism Spectrum Disorder (ASD) and will be able to speak to the autism characteristics and patterns of cognition, specific teaching strategies and program resources. They are able to perform a range of educational assessments to determine specific areas of academics that require attention.

The student (if it is appropriate given the age and/or functioning capacity to participate meaningfully to share personal goals and challenges)

The following is a list of possible key people that you may want to include in an IEP meeting for a student with Autism Spectrum Disorder:

Principal – Principals are legally responsible to ensure that IEPs are in place and being used to facilitate the education of the student. They have access to information regarding staffing and distribution of resources. It is imperative to remember that like a parent, he or she is responsible for making sure that each child in the "family" gets what they need. It is easy to become so focused on one child that we neglect the needs of all children.

A Representative of the school or the school district - Probably a principal or member of administration as these are the people who possess more control over human and material resources than do teachers.

Educational Assistants/Paraprofessionals – The "front line" staff connect daily with the student. They gain first -hand experience with the skills, challenges, and interests of the student. Their observations are critical to the 'whole' picture of where the child is currently and what next steps should be taken.

Guidance Counselors – Educators who may have intricate knowledge about post-secondary or community programs that might be worth considering.

Behaviour Resource Specialist

Autism Spectrum Disorder Consultants

Speech and Language Pathologist, Occupational Therapist, Psychologists - Professionals that know the student well will have gleaned essential insight from the assessments performed with the student. Assessment information needs to be linked to programming and goal setting for the student. Communication, language and sensory concerns cannot be ignored when programming and planning for a student with ASD.

Community Agencies – Some parents will have Case Managers that have helped them to find the proper supports and resources in the community. There can be a level of trust and familiarity between the parent and these people because they have 'been there' through the difficult times. A person from an outside agency may clarify information, ask questions and advocate for the child and parents in a school meeting. They may also add information and insight into the child's world outside of school. This is essential when we are dealing with a student with ASD because program goals need to be generalized (learned in different places, at different times, with different people) if they are to be learned and internalized.

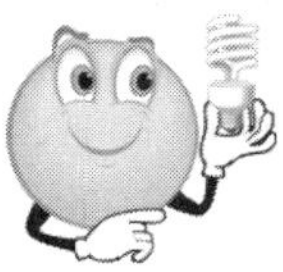

Final Advice from the Front Line

- ✓ Share responsibility; involve key stakeholders.
- ✓ Avoid insisting that other agencies or institutions do things the way you think they should be done. A child's educational meeting is not the place to argue policies and mandates. Be aware that inviting different agencies to a meeting may spark a "clash of mandates" as each group has specific set of skills and mandates. Too often, parents get caught in the cross fire. Tensions increase when one professional tries to 'tell' another what they SHOULD be doing

despite the fact that they may lack the necessary procedural knowledge of that particular institution. For example, a community agency may not have the complete understanding of how money is disbursed for special education students within a school board. The proverbial village will be much more effective when we avoid pointing fingers and take personal responsibility for educating a student. Find another forum to argue about mandates and money!

- ✓ Set time limits and stick to an agenda. Elect someone as the chair of the meeting.
- ✓ Come prepared! Avoid speaking off the top of your head; doing so will run the risk of forgetting important information and/or saying something that is irrelevant or inappropriate. Consider using the Staying on Track During an IEP Meeting template in the Appendices for recording observations and keeping track of what issues need to be addressed.
- ✓ Use personal names of team members not titles when possible (in order to demonstrate equality among participants).
- ✓ Keep notes of the meetings.
- ✓ Ensure that the size of the group is practical. We do not invite people for the purpose of 'stacking' the meeting with a bunch of professionals. People who sit at a meeting need to have excellent knowledge of the child being discussed. The child is central. The child is our reason for being there!
- ✓ Look for common goals. Members should spend time reflecting on the goals, visions and concerns of each member present. Each voice needs to be heard and affirmed, even when we don't agree with parts of the message. We are more likely to work towards solutions when we feel that our ideas are genuinely heard.
- ✓ Listen with the intent of understanding (not responding) and be OPTIMISTIC!

Referral and Assessment

A student can be referred for a special education evaluation by the parent, the teacher or by another professional who is involved with the student. The school must notify the parent that the referral was made and they must get written permission to complete an evaluation. At this point, decisions are made regarding the type of assessments that will be used and the people who will be gathering this information. In the case of autism, it is sensible to ensure that the persons that are doing the assessments are experts in Autism Spectrum Disorders.

Identification and Placement

In the provinces of Canada the process of identifying a student with Autism Spectrum Disorder for the purposes of providing a placement and an appropriate program begins with the formal individual education plan meeting or an Identification Placement Review

Committee Meeting. The name of the process varies from province to province, but, in all cases each child who is not able to access the regular provincial curriculum without extra supports has the legal right to an individualized education plan (IEP). The principal of the school is responsible for organizing this meeting at least once a year, once a student has been identified. The parents must agree on the placement in writing. In cases when parents refuse consent, the reasons for refusal and/or actions undertaken by the school to obtain consent and/or resolve concerns, must be documented. Students in Canada and the United States, will be placed in the most enabling/least restrictive environment. (We still have work to do on that!) This means that, to the greatest extent possible and reasonable, students with autism should be in classes with their peers from the general school population. Students with autism in the U. S. and Canada are placed in a range of settings based on the percentage of time they are outside of the regular education classroom. The range or continuum of placements available to students who have an Autism Spectrum Disorder include:

- a regular classroom
- a resource room
- a separate class
- a separate school
- a residential facility
- the home or a hospital

In selecting an educational setting for a student, the IEP team should consider:

- ✓ The severity of the student's autism
- ✓ The student's need for services that would be related (speech and language, occupational therapy, counseling etc…)
- ✓ The student's ability to adapt to the routines of specific settings
- ✓ The student's need for alternative courses or programs (life skills, vocational training, sensory integration, non-verbal language programs and so on)
- ✓ The student's academic and social skill level
- ✓ The student's age and level of schooling (primary – secondary)

The following is a list of possible placement options:

- Regular classroom with indirect assistance – the student will receive accommodations for learning and assessment in class – no additional resources

- Regular classroom with resource assistance – an educational assistant will be available to (not attached to) the student on a full time or part time basis

- Regular classroom with withdrawal assistance – the student will be part time in a regular class and part time outside of it.

- Special Education class with partial integration – the student will spend part of his time in a regular class or in a social setting with typical students (Physical Education, Learning for Living, Technology Class, Art/Music, Vocational training etc.)

❖ Special Education class full time – this placement requires that the committee state valid reasons why this placement is a best fit for the student with autism.

Components of an Individual Education Plan

- ✓ Student identification/profile
- ✓ Special services and supports that are required (specialized equipment and professional support)
- ✓ Recent assessment dates
- ✓ Current levels of performance (agreed upon by the team) and stated for each subject area
- ✓ Student strengths and areas of need in terms of skills
- ✓ General accommodations for all subject areas
- ✓ Student specific learning goals (both academic and functional)
- ✓ Performance objectives (must be very specific and measurable)
- ✓ Core teaching strategies
- ✓ A statement of the methods that will be used to assess and measure the achievement of goals and the timelines that will be followed.
- ✓ A statement that explains to what extent the student will not be participating with general education students in regular class activities
- ✓ Names of personnel who will implement the education plan and the location where it will be implemented
- ✓ Plans for evaluation and review (specify dates)
- ✓ Plans for activities and services that will facilitate transition from secondary school into the community, postsecondary and/or workplace (must be in place by the age of 16 and updated annually)

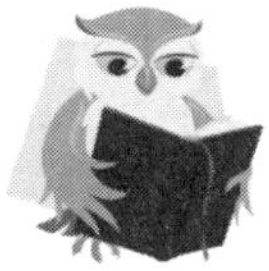

"Planning is bringing the future into the present so that you can do something about it now."

Alan Lakein

Show Me The Blueprints Please!

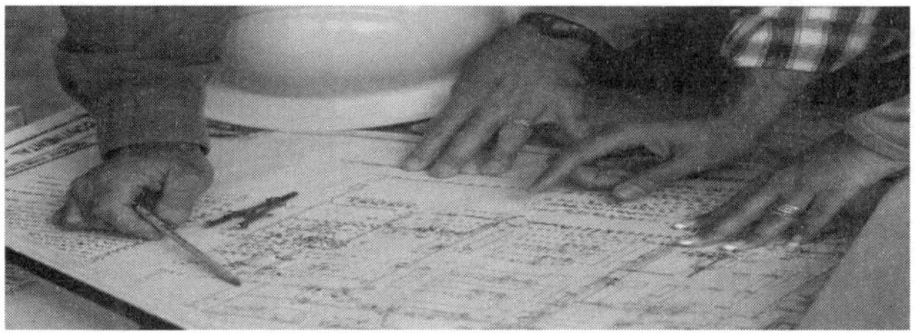

Everything worth doing is worth planning

Overview of the Process

1) Gathering Information: Making use of Students Records, School history, Medical History and Assessments
2) The Blueprint
3) Integrating a Transition Plan
4) Implementing the IEP: Keeping it Real
5) Assessment Drives Instruction

1) Gathering Information: Making use of Students Records, School History, Medical History and Assessments

The next step is to begin to compile relevant information that will help lead the team to decisions about where the child is at academically and functionally and where they envision him or her to be at the end of the school year. The following is a list of the human and material resources that are helpful in gathering information. Remember that the whole child needs to be represented and each piece of information adds to the whole picture.

Student records: report cards, professional reports, relevant medical information, previous education plan meetings, information regarding specialized equipment or health services

Professional assessments: For example: Psychological Assessments, Standardized Achievement Tests, Speech and Language Pathologist, and Occupational Therapist assessments, Educational assessments). Be sure to look for areas of strength that could be harnessed to develop weak skills. These assessments are not to be used as “proof” that there is no point in skill building because test scores are bleak

Parents: Parents have key information that will help to prioritize goals and objectives.

Previous teachers: It is advantageous to discuss strategies, resources and methods that worked in the past and those that were not helpful. It is unfair to the child if each teacher needs to use trial and error to learn what works and what doesn’t

Educational Assistants: The "front line" staff who have daily contact with the student and firsthand experience of the skills, challenges and interests of the student. If they cannot be present at the meeting, their input should be recorded in writing and presented at the meeting.

Samples of student work: If available, this is evidence of the student's skill and performance level. Samples provide information about strengths, needs and the child's rate of progress. Portfolios of student work demonstrate where the student has been in certain skill areas and where the team should aim to direct him in skill development.

CAUTION

> **An overarching principle of any IEP is that there must be a logical connection which flows from assessment information to the strengths and needs, accommodations/modifications, goals/objectives, teaching strategies and assessment methods. This connection makes the IEP authentic and worthwhile.**

Different provinces, territories and states will host different formats (just to keep it fun) and so the sample provided is not definitive. It is an example that will hopefully demonstrate the different components of goal setting and the 'building plan.'

2) The Blueprint

Strengths and Needs

Always start with the positives when discussing a student. Few people are inspired by having a list of their deficits stated with little effort but their assets require contemplation or worse – creative thought! Construct an educational plan with the foundation of skills and abilities the student possesses. What skills can we draw on to build the areas of need? For example, if the student has a strong visual learning style we should use it to help compensate for a weaker auditory style.

The list that follows is a general smorgasbord of strengths and needs that could describe a student. Specific goals will be listed later in the book. When choosing which skills to record, make sure that they are REAL and not what you or anybody else would like to believe! I have added some explanations for the sake of clarification of educational jargon. And one more thing - describe skills and learning styles, not personality characteristics, to list strengths and needs!

- Visual spatial skills – the ability to process information primarily in pictures/images rather than words; ideas are interconnected (imagine a web) rather than in a linear sequence - Some visual-spatial learners are excellent at auditory sequential processing as well

- Metacognitive skills - the ability to reflect on one's own thinking process
- Expressive language skills – about half of children with ASD have a severe language delay- with early intervention the majority of children with autism will improve language skills
- Receptive language skills – the ability to understand what others are saying – not to just hear them but to 'get the message'
- Time management skills – deciding how long to work on one assignment and leaving time to complete others
- Visual memory skills – remembering what you have seen exactly as it was
- Oral language skills – the ability to use sophisticated vocabulary and grammar, accurate pronunciation, to effectively express oneself in his or her social environment
- Reading comprehension skills – understanding the message of what is being read
- Basic reading and decoding skills – able to read words and/or sound them out without necessarily understanding them
- Problem solving skills –looking at the components of a problem, deciding which steps will lead to a solution; considering potential options
- Articulation skills- speaking clearly and creating the proper sounds specific to letter combinations
- Self- advocacy skills – the ability to describe your own needs – example, "Please slow down when you speak to me. I need time to understand what you are saying."
- Visual – motor learning skills – eye-hand coordination
- Conversational skills – ability to initiate a conversation, take turns in speaking and transition to new topics as the conversation flows
- Anxiety management skills – ability to recognize when one is anxious and use a strategy or a tool to cope
- Communication skills – both verbal and non -verbal ways of letting someone know thoughts, feelings, ideas
- Adaptive behaviour skills – independent living skills (self-care, managing a home, being a consumer, living in a community etc...)
- Rote memory skills – too often this is mistaken for true understanding of a concept – a student who can count from 1 to 100 does not necessarily know the meaning of the value of a number

- Computing skills – the ability to calculate numbers without using paper, pencil or calculator (as in the case of Dustin Hoffman in the movie Rain Man); again, be aware, that computing skills do not necessarily mean that the student has an understanding of money values or number values
- Mathematical problem solving and reasoning – using math concepts to solve abstract math problems
- Organizational skills – the ability to manage time, materials, and space efficiently
- Written language skills – the ability to organize one's thoughts mentally, record and present them in a structured coherent way (with proper spelling, mechanics and grammar)
- Spelling, punctuation and capitalization rules
- Auditory skills – one who learns by actively listening to the sounds in the environment (actually listening to what one hears and being able to understand)
- Auditory memory skills – the ability to store what you hear and recall it when you need it (telephone numbers, multi -step instructions)
- Auditory sequencing skills – the ability to remember the order of items in a list such as the alphabet, months, days, numbers
- Visual skills – the ability to learn and organize ideas that are seen
- Self -help skills – dressing, toileting, hygiene, preparing meals, eating with utensils
- Computer skills – the ability to use the keyboard and programs to create a product, web page or layout or simple
- Keyboarding skills
- Sequential skills – knowing how to put pictures or words in an order that is logical
- Sensory regulation skills – being able to regulate some of their own sensory issues and to communicate a sensory need
- Self -regulation skills - involves controlling behaviour, goal-setting, self-monitoring, time management and organization, study and learning strategies, and test-taking strategies
- Social language skills – also known as pragmatics – eye contact, turn taking in conversation, personal space etc...
- Fine motor skills - small muscle movements such as those used in printing, cutting, colouring etc…
- Gross Motor skills – large muscle movements such as those used in jumping, running, throwing a ball etc…

- Building, repair or assembling things
- Drawing skills or creating art

The list of needs on an IEP should not be dramatically longer than the list of strengths for a student. Keep in mind that if you list an area of need, it would make sense that you are ready and willing to address it in the IEP and the student's programming. The IEP includes what will be assessed, not all that will be taught during the term.

What are Accommodations and Modifications? What IS the Difference?

Accommodations are:

- Changes made to the teaching strategies that will allow a student with Autism Spectrum Disorder to learn the regular curriculum.
- Changes made to the classroom or school environment for the student to be able to access the curriculum.
- Changes made to assessment practices that will allow a student to demonstrate learning of regular curriculum.

Accommodations do not require specified goals and measurable outcomes in the education plan.

While many accommodations are considered just 'good teaching', they are often critical for the success of a student with autism. Well -chosen accommodations build a bridge so that the student has the opportunity to achieve goals within the curriculum. Imagine how prosthetics give a child the ability to walk and run. No one would consider that prosthetics are a 'crutch' to the child; the child would not somehow be motivated to walk without them. The same can be said about our use of accommodations that help to make up for some of the neurological challenges faced by children with autism.

I think sometimes we don't take accommodations seriously enough. Our mindset as educators must be focus on findings ways for students to be able to learn and to demonstrate learning. We offer accommodations to help accomplish just that. They do not guarantee a student's success (or lack of failure), but set up equity -- a level playing field.

Instructional Accommodations

- While teaching, provide an external structure to lessons through a written outline of the main points to be learned
- Make use of visual supports such as personal daily schedules, first -then boards, social stories, charts, graphic organizers
- Incorporate pictures, images and other visual aids when teaching vocabulary words, scientific subjects and abstract concepts
- Provide varying levels of prompts (verbal, physical, gesture, visual)

- Provide more opportunities to repeat and practice a skill in another setting, with different materials and people (teach skill to another student)
- Break down steps and skills into smaller units
- Use visual materials (Time Timers™, notes, schedules) to prepare for changes in routine and transitions (except in emergencies)
- Use modeling ina small group or one to one situation to demonstrate a new skill (it helps to show a finished product as well)
- Write instructions in clear, sequential, short steps
- Pair verbal instructions with written format
- List assignments or steps of an assignment in a checklist format and check - in with student throughout the process
- Opportunity to work in a quiet area especially when new concepts are introduced
- Explicitly teach and explain how and why the concept being taught is useful (autistic students can't infer this level of understanding intuitively)
- Leave NOTHING implied or assumed…spell out exactly what is expected in concrete terms
- Provide 'wait time' for processing
- Use word retrieval prompts
- Teach the use of time management aids (alarms, digital reminders)
- Use augmentative and alternative communications systems
- Avoid expecting notes to be copied from board
- Extra time for assignments with check - in points
- Arrange a signal with a student to indicate you will be asking a question of him soon or provide the question before class (reduces anxiety) so he can prepare
- Reinforcement may be needed to increase motivation to complete assignments that are less intrinsically rewarding or interesting
- Limit homework and make sure that it is just drill or repetition of a skill already taught; no new skills
- Incorporate relaxation techniques into the student's schedule (deep breathing, Snoezelen™ Room/sensory room, water breaks, listening to music etc…)
- Dramatize information (see episodic memory)
- Provide duplicated notes

<u>Writing:</u>

- Allow the student to use a word processing program whenever possible
- Oral discussion of ideas prior to writing
- Provide 2 or 3 topics if brainstorming is challenging for the student
- Provide graphic organizers for developing ideas in an organized, visual format
- Scribe when written output is overwhelming
- One to one assistance with editing
- Provide a slant board to compensate for vestibular problems (a binder works well as well)
- Allow the student to use a vibrating pen, weighted pen, felt tip pen
- Provide the student with raised lined paper to increase proprioceptive input to cue for line usage (this also works with vertical margins)
- Allow the student to write about favourite topics whenever possible

- Use a tape recorder to record answers or responses rather than a written format (See Assistive Technology Guide in the Appendices)

Math:

- Use concrete manipulatives to teach and reinforce concepts (clocks, learning carpets, tangrams, attribute blocks etc…)
- Step by step instruction with visual cues
- Use of number chart and calculator for problem solving
- Reduction of repetitive problems
- Regular review and drill even after moving to a new concept
- Provide a quiet area or small group instruction to learn new skills
- Expand a word problem to a higher copy ratio (150%) so that the student is able to cut out the extra, irrelevant information and arrange the important words and symbols
- Provide a "cheat sheet" of symbols and words (sum means add, less than means subtract)

Reading:

- Use visual maps for sequencing beginning, middle and end
- Use graphic organizers to outline the elements of stories (characters, plot, setting, problem, solution)
- Use computer software to the child
- Explain idioms, metaphor and satire explicitly (do not assume that the student understands)
- Provide immediate feedback directly to student throughout long texts or assignments
- Use visuals (arrows, boxes, highlights) to help students to focus on important points and key words
- Give the student the questions before he begins reading

Environmental Accommodations:

- Provide an external structure to the school day by posting a visual schedule of the subjects and events of the day
- Provide softer lighting in the classroom or turn off fluorescent lights when possible
- Provide a 'safe spot' or a break card (if possible decide with the student a place in the classroom where he or she may retreat to in times of increasing stimulation or if overwhelmed)
- Consider sensory sensitivities and possible distractions when choosing where to seat the student within the classroom
- Visual cues to stay on task (visual clocks, picture symbols, gesture)
- Tennis balls on the legs of chairs to reduce noise
- Provide earplugs and teach the student when to use them
- Allow personal music devices (MP3 player, ipod) with classical or soothing music

- Logical layout of materials and resources; clearly defined areas for specific tasks and activities
- Clutter-free bulletin boards and shelf space so as to highlight only important information (context)
- Sensory diet tools and activities are in a clearly marked and accessible area
- Allow a student to enter class a few minutes early and leave a few minutes late in order to avoid the chaos of the hallways during class change

Assessment and Evaluation Accommodations:

- Demonstrate skill in learning style that student is strongest in example: performance of skill, visual exhibit, oral report, matching responses, choosing from multiple responses, pointing to correct answer, Yes/No etc...
- Provide the student with a written outline of the material that will be covered on the test
- Change the format of question (oral instead of written)
- Allow extra time (some assessments may need to be scheduled over several class periods or days)
- Reduce the amount of questions or tasks
- Frequent breaks
- Provide a choice for demonstration of the skill
- Use of augmentative communication system as used in non-evaluative activities
- Allow the student to use a word processing computer program whenever possible
- Provide an alternative setting that is quiet with fewer students
- Highlight the directions to the test so that the student will focus on them
- List page numbers of important sections of a book to help the student study
- Consider objective style responses such as multiple choice and short answer rather than essay style responses
- Allow the student to actively move during assessments (stand up to write, walk, jump, chew gum, hold a squishy ball or have a Theraband ™ on the chair legs)

Alternative Programs or Courses

Given the range of areas affected by autism it is not surprising that the educational plan of students with ASD may include partial or whole alternative programming. Alternative programs or courses describe learning outside of provincial/territorial/state standards and curriculum. Courses relate directly to the specific needs of the learner (as identified on the formal and informal assessments). Examples would be speech and language remediation by a speech pathologist or a special education teacher, social skills training, non- verbal language programs, self –regulation training, occupational therapy lessons and activities and vocational training.

Modifications

Accommodations change HOW a student accesses information and demonstrates learning; modifications change WHAT a student is expected to learn. Both are based on identified needs from the assessment information.

Modifications consist of changing the amount or the complexity of the regular curriculum. Modifications may include using expectations from a lower (or higher) grade level or significantly reducing the number of expectations. In high school, students usually work towards achieving the grade level expectations in the pathway or stream they have chosen: non-credit, locally developed, applied or academic. Choosing the best fitted stream will generally address their learning needs. If the principal approves, there can be changes in number or level of difficulty of the grade level expectations. If a student in secondary is not able to meet expectations at grade level this usually means they are not in the appropriate pathway. A principal will usually not grant a credit if expectations are significantly different for a student.

Educators must be mindful that the extent to which we modify the grade level expectations may change the course of the student's life by closing doors later in his or her school career. Modifications should never be taken lightly or made without consulting members of the student's team: the classroom teacher, special education teacher, parents and sometimes the principal. Elementary school teachers carry an enormous ethical burden: the choices we make in a students' younger years can affect the course of his or her life.

Looking back, it would have been much easier on us, the teachers, support staff and our son if we had simply modified the expectations from the core subjects to a curriculum from a lower grade level. We were reluctant to do so until we had consistently implemented the accommodations he needed and adapted our teaching to match his learning style. I use the word 'we' because I too, was his classroom teacher in both Kindergarten and grade three! I was living the challenge of walking my talk! If we had jumped to modification of core subjects in his elementary years the decision would have made it much more complicated for him to enter university level courses in high school. Instead, the team became creative as to how we could best support his learning with systematic accommodations and some alternative programming, leaving the door open to higher level courses later on.

As I sat at grade 12 graduation ceremonies this year, I was struck by how those decisions earlier in his life left doors open to post-secondary studies. In elementary school his autism severely impacted our son. We had no way of knowing that higher level education would be a possibility. Our son was not "cured." But, he taught me that judgments and assumptions regarding another's ability or disability is dangerous and grossly unfair. Each person can and will grow – given a team or village who will plan today's learning with tomorrow's needs in mind. Always two steps ahead and always believing that our students are gifts.

For each subject modified, the annual goals, current level of performance, specific objectives, resources, assessment methods and timelines must be recorded. This is not the case for accommodations. Students can have both accommodations and modifications on their IEP.

Present Level of Performance

After deciding which modifications will best support the student, the next step will be to record the **Present Level of Performance** (also called the Current Level of Performance) for specific subjects to be modified. Depending on your jurisdiction or school board these statements may be short and sweet or quite descriptive. It is best to check with a special education specialist in your area to determine the wording and detail your administration expects.

This statement must reflect how the student's current strengths and weaknesses (both academic performance and functional performance) affect his or her involvement and progress in the regular provincial curriculum. The intention is that this statement will be comprehensive and objective enough to provide baseline data from which a clear indication of where the skills must be further developed. The planning team must look at examining what a student can do in each subject area of need and then create a goal and objective that links the present level of performance to that goal.

Johnny's echolalia impacts his ability to participate in social educational settings where he is required to respond when asked "wh" questions (group work, board games). He requires prompts to limit repetition and respond consistently.

Notice how the current level reflects the student's expressive language difficulties, his echolalia and gives direction as to what the goals and objectives should be?

Mary's executive function deficits impact her ability to participate in mainstream educational settings that do not provide visual organizers and step by step instructions. She has significant difficulty planning projects, writing essays and following verbal instructions.

Beth's sensory issues make it difficult for her to access the general curriculum when she is not provided with a daily sensory diet. She has significant difficulty attending to what is important and regulating her behaviour and emotions.

Bob's difficulty with critical thinking impacts his ability to predict how a character will respond in a story without partner brainstorming and discussion using visual supports such as Comic Strip Conversations.™

Some levels of performance are more easily quantified:

Billy is able to identify and read 50 out of 200 Basic Sight Vocabulary Words from the Oelwein list consistently 9 out of 10 times.

Maggie is able to accurately skip count by 2's and 5's to fifty 9 out of 10 times. She has not yet demonstrated the ability to count by 2's and 5's to one hundred

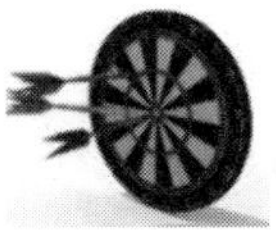

Setting Authentic Goals for Students With Autism

Students need **SMART** goals. Students with autism need **SMARTER** goals! Goals must state a skill or action that the student will be realistically able to achieve in a school year.

S = Specific - name exactly what would be seen if the goal was being met

M = Measurable – identify concrete criteria that can be counted

A = Action – start with a verb that shows what the student will <u>do</u>

R = Realistic –reflect the reality of the student's unique learning style/needs

T = Timely – bound by a time limit so that demonstration of the skill can be

E = Everywhere – skills learned must be carried out in many settings in order to promote generalization

R = Repeated –achieved goals must be maintained over months/years (may also need more repetitions to gain mastery of a skill)

Measures of Success: How do We Measure Skills?

The best goals are those that are specific, measurable, active, realistic and bound by time. The methods most often used to quantify skill progress starts with collecting baseline data. This measure tells what a student is doing before we apply any intervention or teaching. To measure baseline data and skill acquisition educators use a variety of tools:

- Formal assessment tools (implemented by the Special Education Teacher, Speech and Language Pathologist, Psychologist, Occupational Therapist etc...)
- Tally sheets that show a specific number of times per day
- Specific amounts of time (7 minutes, 10 minutes etc...)
- Fractions of time that a skill will be demonstrated (5 minutes out of 20 minutes)
- Percentages of trials, distances, accuracy, and frequency (especially when we are looking for the mastering of a skill 80 -90% of trials)
- Levels of prompts (always working towards fading the prompt levels and moving towards the most independence possible)

One concern is that too often when a skill can't be quantified it is not written as a goal for "fear" of not including a measurement component. For example, how do we measure the use of social cues, social language, self -monitoring, impulse control and more 'implicit' skills?

There are times when it is necessary to use qualitative "measurements" of skills that are not easily calculable. Consider the fact that The Diagnostic Statistical Manual (DSM) describes autism in terms of its "qualitative impairments." Sometimes we cannot quantify expectations but that does not diminish their significance.

Educational teams could discuss and agree on Qualitative Scales that describe the quality of the behaviour or skill in levels. Teachers do this when assessing story writing, written work, drama roles and problem solving. Use levels and rubrics to describe a baseline and goals for achievement. What qualities need to be observed? What observable behaviours will be seen to reflect growth in a skill area?

It is also imperative to delineate the skills with a task analysis: break down the action or skill into the steps that are necessary. Identify the steps in the skill and the level of prompt/support. Data can be taken from the observation of each step.

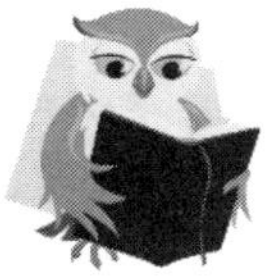

> ***What you get by achieving your goals is not as important as what you become by achieving your goals.***
>
> ***Goethe***

Using Prompt Levels and Generalization as Measure of Success

What is a Prompt?

Have you ever been in a play and had the unfortunate experience of forgetting your lines? And then, like an angel from heaven, a voice in the wings whispered the words that were failing you? Likewise, parents too, prompt their children to remember their manners: "What's the magic word?" We use prompts to give additional information so that success and/ or a correct response is more likely.

Using prompts is really not rocket science! But, when using prompts to teach skills and increase independence with students with autism it does become more of an art. Effective prompts are delivered *immediately* after a question or instruction and before the response is given. The whole point of prompting is to activate a correct response before a student can make an error. Errors are very hard to 'unteach.'

The key to successful prompting is in *prompt fading*. Just as a baby needs to eventually be weaned from a bottle or a pacifier, prompts need to be faded for students. When teaching a new skill prompt levels need to become less and less intrusive. For example, taking a child's hand and leading him across the street eventually becomes a gesture or a nod to look both ways and eventually walking side by side with no cues. We do this naturally with typical children because it would be quite a sight to see a mother leading her grown son across the street! We need to be more vigilant about fading our cues with autistic children as well. Sometimes in the name of 'helping' a student we are actually crippling his or her ability to develop autonomy!

The following are prompts in the order of most intrusive to least, usually used to teach a NEW skill:

Verbal – Additional information given (not the same as the original instruction). "What is next? Check your schedule. Sit down. Stand up." Much like nagging – and we all know how effective that is!

Physical – hand over hand, holding hands (can also be a partial physical such as guiding a person's hand, or wrist to the correct response

Model – demonstration of each step of task

Gesture - pointing, nodding, using our face to communicate yes or no

Positional - the target item (or correct response) is placed in a location that is closer to the child

Visual – pictures, written lists, visual schedules – anything visual that gives additional information needed to complete a task or learn a skill

When teaching a new skill, we need to be sure that the student will learn the 'correct' way to complete the task the first time. We may start with a full physical prompt but we gradually reduce our role in carrying out the task. Think of a child learning to ride a bicycle: the parent gradually releases their grasp of the bike until the child is riding independently.

The most difficult prompts to fade are those that we do not even know we are using. Taking a coat off of the hanger, turning on the tap, gazing towards the correct answer, forming the beginning of the words with our mouths and even changing our facial expression when the child is close to the correct response are all prompts that may go undetected. But, if not faded, these simple actions could leave the student with autism unable to respond in the prompts absence. Autism has a nasty way of convincing kids that our unconscious cues are part of the steps required to execute an action.

Lastly, individuals on the autism spectrum tend to work in one sensory mode at a time. If we are giving directions and expecting the student to write at the same time it probably won't happen because an autistic brain is not wired to multitask. The same can be said for asking for eye contact while learning thinking of a response to a question. We have to be very careful that we are not "overloading" the sensory channels when we expect a student to respond to us.

What is Generalization?

Once a skill or a step has been taught and practiced so thoroughly that a student is able to perform the task without any prompts (and on different days) the skill is said to be mastered. But, mastery is not the last step when we teach a student with autism. We have to help the student to be able to complete the task or the step in different places, at various times and with other people. This step is critical because as we learned in the Cognitive section of this book, individuals with autism do not automatically use a learned skill in new situations. Instead, the autistic brain tends to learn information in isolation, failing to see the most relevant resemblance between tasks or actions. Thus, for a student with autism, learning to use a skill in different rooms or situations, with a variety of materials and/or people requires explicit teaching on the part of educators. This is true for high functioning individuals with autism as well.

Personally, I learned about generalization problems the hard way. After many months of skateboarding lessons in an indoor skate park by a trained instructor my husband thought Kieran would enjoy using his new skills at a local outdoor skate park. Upon arrival at the park, our 11 year old son was despondent. When questioned as to what was wrong, he informed his dad that he hadn't learned how to skateboard at this park! Both returned home frustrated with the other. The only way we could convince Kieran that he did in fact have the skills he needed, was to hire a "skate buddy/instructor" to "re-teach" the already learned skills at various parks in the city. Up until that point, the skill hadn't been generalized.

Telling time on only one clock, using only the toilet at home, using one type calculator, and doing multiplication only at your desk are other potential glaring generalization snags. In high school, learning that the scientific method can be used beyond the science class and that the graphic organizer used for writing an English essay will likely work in Geography are examples of the need for explicit generalization. These connections will not be made intuitively for our kids with autism. The generalization step is extremely important for all kinds of academic and functional life skills.

To be sure that skills are truly learned, generalization plans need to be embedded into the teaching plan and into the IEP. It is not good enough that the student is able to recite his or her name and address to the classroom teacher; the skill will have to be practiced with other staff, at home and in the community before we can say with any confidence that the student can do it independently!

Rallying the help of custodians, secretaries, administrators and volunteers in the school is the easiest way to teach generalization. When students have mastered a skill in a direct teaching structure it is imperative that they be expected to use their new skills in more natural settings. For example, counting change could be extended from the student desk to counting change in another classroom and eventually to counting change for the parent volunteers on pizza day. It takes planning and cooperation of others, but, incorporating generalization procedures into the goal planning makes a student's learning relevant and real.

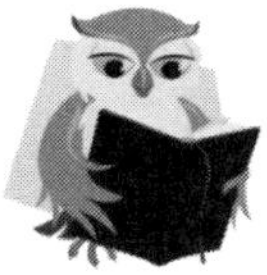

> ***When goals go, meaning goes.***
> ***When meaning goes, purpose goes.***
> ***When purpose goes,***
> ***Life goes dead on our hands.***
> ***Carl Jung***

Annual Goals: The Big Picture

Goals are global in nature. Goals reflect what the parents, student and educational team target as important skills to be learned and used by the end of the school year. Goals are derived from assessment data. Goals for "autism curriculum" such as self - regulation, emotional development and so on can be embedded within state or provincial curriculum. These can also stand alone as alternative programming.

The specific formats for the recording of goals will vary according to educational jurisdictions. But, the essence of individual planning remains the same – set meaningful, realistic goals, based on the student's needs and measure progress consistently in order to modify the program to fit the child.

Choosing goals: Think **global**, **functional**, **relevant** and **developmental**

1. What is the most meaningful content for the development of the student?

Do your homework: Use information to determine exactly what the student needs. What is essential that the child learn? (Is it *really* going to advance his independence and wellbeing if he can name all the states or provinces?)

What possibilities exist for future goals (high school, post -secondary, supported living, and employment)? BE CAREFUL

2. How will autism needs be addressed?

Consider language, social skills, self- regulation, emotional understanding, sensory needs and executive function skills, working memory. Avoid focusing solely on "behaviour management" because there is a very good chance that by addressing other areas of need, behaviour problems will diminish.

3. Are the skills developmentally appropriate?

What can the student do? What is the next developmental step? If a student is not successful examine the developmental scope and sequence of the skill and seriously consider the child's zone of proximal development - are you teaching "in the window?" We cannot expect a student to learn how to count coins if he is struggling with identifying the value of coins (1 nickel equals 5 pennies). If the student has not yet gained an ability to think in the abstract, learning the states of matter or the geographical regions of the world may not be very useful.

- **Global**: What can be accomplished in a year?
- **Functional**: based on the student's needs
- **Relevant:** for the future development of the student's learning and independence?
- **Developmental:** realistic given current functioning

I must also confess that it is much easier to write a broad goal full of attitudes and beliefs than it is a SMART goal. Let me show you what I mean:

VAGUE GOAL

Mary will develop friendship skills. *(Why hasn't she already? What is her problem?)*

While friendship skills are lovely the goal doesn't answer some critical questions.

Who?

Will do what?

Under what conditions?

In what time frame?

To what level or degree?

How will progress be measured?

Let's attempt to make this goal a SMART goal:

Mary will improve her ability to play interactively with a classmate. Using visual supports to take turns, she will play a board game with a peer 3 times per week for a one month period. Mary will increase the frequency of waiting her turn (without hitting herself or crying) from 0 times per game to 10 times per game or the equivalent of 90% of the time.

VAGUE GOAL

Thomas will stay seated in class. (Poor Thomas, will he ever be able to get up?)

SMARTER GOAL

Using picture rehearsal, a Time Timer™ and reinforcement, Thomas will increase his time on-task during independent written seat work from 1 minute to 10 minutes at three different points during the school day for three consecutive weeks.

VAGUE GOAL

Bill will learn fractions.

SMARTER GOAL

By the end of the year, Bill will demonstrate an understanding of basic fractions by matching written fractions with the correct amounts of a variety of items with 90% accuracy over the course of three assessment probes. (I.e. match the numbers ¼ with a ¼ piece of play pizza, chocolate bar, Cuisenaire rods and so on).

Note: an assessment probe is simply a point during the school year in which a quick redo of the skill is done with the student to ensure it has been maintained accurately.

In my work with families I see all kinds of vague goals: goals that are meaningless (big on promise, short on specifics). What gets me bothered the most, is when goals seem to depict the child as the problem; the child just needs to get his act together and then all would be well! Equally as useless, are goals that are attitudinal statements. We cannot measure an attitude as it is an internal state of mind. Goals that fail to give specific information are not worth the time they take to be written. How effective would you consider these goals?

I will lose weight.
I will get good grades.
I will eat healthy food.

Consider the following educational goals:

Demonstrate an understanding that school is a safe place.
Commitment to academic success.
Develop healthy peer relationships.
Be a good friend.
Complete all of the grade 3 reading expectations.
Be more organized in her school work.

The examples are noble goals, but they lack the specifics that will transform them from lofty intentions into practical and achievable goals. Does this sound more achievable?

I will eat one boiled egg for a morning snack, one cup of vegetables with my lunch and dinner, 5 days a week for three months.

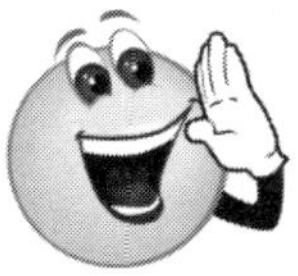

Writing goals is directly reflective of the student's present level of performance. The measures that are provided in the sample are obviously arbitrary numbers based on imagined baseline data. It is CRITICAL that staff collect baseline data: the behaviour or skill is measured before an intervention is applied so that the amount of progress can be quantified or qualified.

Specific Performance Objectives

Specific Performance Expectations/Objectives are more precise because they break down the global annual goal into attainable steps. Each goal contains **sub-skills** that must be taught in a logical sequence so that the student is able to internalize the concept and generalize the skill. Specific expectations may also reflect the need to increase independence in skill acquisition by **decreasing the level of prompt**s provided. The short term objectives MUST be based on the annual goals which MUST relate to the student's present level of performance.

- Analyze the annual goal into sequential, intermediate steps that lead to reaching it.
- MUST be based on the annual goals which MUST relate to the student's present level of performance.
- What indicators of progress toward meeting the goal will be measured intermittently during the year?

Goal

Objective 1:	Objective 2:	Objective 3:
first step towards goal	2nd step towards goal	third step towards goal

Developing specific objectives step by step:

1. Choose **one skill** at a time.
2. Decide the **level of support** that is going to be provided (prompt levels and type of prompts) based on the current level of performance.
3. Write each expectation to reflect the **incremental steps** towards independent functioning of the skill.
4. Choose the **context** or setting that the skill will be learned.
5. Record the **criteria** that will be used to measure success (mastery of the skill).
6. Include the expectation for **generalization** of the skill.
7. Set the learning **time frame** one term/semester.

Example Goal:

When working on independent learning tasks in the classroom, Owen will independently transition from one activity to another by interacting with a Do/Done Visual Board for all of his independent tasks in a school day. Progress will be monitored by staff recording whether the activity is completed and the task card moved from DO to DONE position.

Mastery criteria will be at least 4 out of 5 task cards moved and task completion for 5 days for two consecutive weeks. Owen will demonstrate generalization by independently completing this skill in math class, language arts and during physical education.

Corresponding Objectives:

1. With *full physical prompts*, Owen will go to the schedule after completion of an independent learning task, remove the task picture from the "DO" position and place it on the "Done" column for 3 out of 5 tasks once a day for two weeks.

2. With *non- verbal prompts and partial physical prompts*, Owen will go to the schedule after completion of an independent learning task, remove the task picture from the "DO" position and place it on the "Done" column for 5 out of 5 tasks in the math and again during *physical education*.

3. With only the *visual prompt* of the task schedule, Owen will independently transition from one independent learning task, remove the task picture from the "DO" position and place it on the "Done" column and proceed to the next task on 5 out of 5 tasks in *math, language arts* and again during *physical education every day for two weeks.*

I realize that this example is "meaty." I purposely included a lot of information in order to make the point that we often leave too many specifics out of the IEP. This could be why we fail to see progress. When teaching students with autism, the steps towards achieving a goal may be much smaller than they are for a typical learner. Real progress gets hidden when the steps are too large.

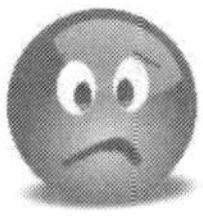

Please DON'T!

- Use general terms such as "appropriate behaviour", "making good progress," "earned good grades"
- Use value judgements such as "degree of effort"
- Pull goals out of... the air
- Repeat the same goals and objectives year after year
- Use the same criteria and the same method of assessment for every goal

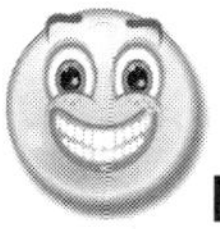

Please DO

- Incorporate incremental prompt levels and fading into objectives
- Share progress data sheets and/or graphs with parents and student often
- Involve parents and student in the drafting of goals
- Incorporate self -monitoring whenever possible
- Report on observations and facts – not attitudes and values
- If it's in the IEP...DO IT!

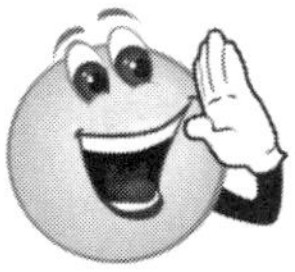

Students with autism WILL progress when programs, resources and goals are matched to their unique needs and strengths.

As much as I would love to be able to offer a menu of program goals that teachers and parents could pick and choose from, I think that that would be far beyond the scope of one book and that it would be too much like a "drop down" menu" on an educational software program. I detest those because they are too generic!

CAUTION

The following list of goals and objectives **do not** demonstrate the SMART description of the goal. The purpose of this listing of possible goals and objectives is to demonstrate the wide range of potential areas for programming and the autism specific needs that must be met.

In choosing this "smorgasbord" approach I have broken several cardinal rules of writing educational plans: The goals and objectives are generic and they do not match each other! The goals are not written to answer ALL of these questions. Please keep this in mind as you review the following lists. They are provided as a starting place.

Who? Will do what? Under what conditions? In what time frame? To what degree or level? How will progress be monitored?

In addition, if you are to use a goal or objective from this list, it must reflect your student's needs. In addition, be sure to either **break down the goal** into manageable sub -skills, varying prompt levels, gradients of success or percentages of successful trials. You might also **build up the objective** from its sub-skills to a broader goal by increasing the expectation of independence, the number of accurate responses, the quality of responses and/or the percentage of accuracy.

Social Communication and Language Goals

A trained Speech and Language Pathologist should be guiding the goal setting of the language and communication domains whenever it is possible. Communication is one of the core deficits in autism and it makes sense that programming needs be based on recent and ongoing assessment. This is not to say that a teacher or a paraprofessional cannot deliver the program set up by a speech specialist. The speech of many students with autism is impacted by dyspraxia and a qualified Speech and Language Pathologist (SLP) should outline instructional techniques and goals.

But as we know, social communication goes far beyond the ability to speak. Receptive and expressive language, pragmatics, perspective taking and a host of other skills are involved. Students with autism will need direct and systematic teaching of social communication within and outside of the state or provincial curriculum. It is crucial that we help students develop the ability to think and interact socially and flexibly over time. These are not skills that we teach once and then move on. Initially, we may have to teach directly in small group or one to one setting. The critical aspect of social skills development is that we extend and monitor the skills learned to more natural environments. Group work, clubs and daily interactions become the "practicum" component of training.

Measuring social communication with numbers and percentages may be too contrived and less meaningful in real life settings. I have found that success rubrics that demonstrate qualitative descriptions of the outward signs of social success are the most helpful for teachers and students. Self- monitoring is greatly enhanced when we create qualitative scales and rubrics with the student.

The time limits recorded in the examples below are intended to demonstrate that a time restriction and observable behaviour is necessary for a goal to be SMARTER. Remember you have to be able to see the behaviour that you are describing. We cannot measure attitudes.

- ☑ Student will increase his ability to communicate by independently exchanging pictures for desired items/activities. Upon seeing and wanting a particular item and with a picture of that item <u>in reach</u>, student will pick up the picture, reach to the person holding the item, and release the picture into that person's hand. He will <u>independently</u> complete request sequence without prompts for 4 of 5 opportunities when trainer is in close proximity (within 1 foot).
- ☑ Using Clicker 5 program, student will answer correctly 2 of each "w" questions (who, what, when, and where) that are relevant to his life with no prompting on 5 non- consecutive days.
- ☑ Correctly label (receptively) 30 pictures of food items 9 out of 10 times at three probes during the course of the year (December, March and May).
- ☑ Correctly and independently respond to yes/no questions presented randomly 9 out of 10 times at three probes during the course of the year (December, March and May).
- ☑ By the end of the school year, student will use a Voice Output Device to request a preferred activity without any prompting from staff.
- ☑ Using a verbal prompt, "Do this" student will mirror the actions of others involving the manipulation of physical objects. He will perform the imitation response 8 out of 10 times with no physical prompts at his work table.
- ☑ By the end of the year, student will actively participate as member of the "Fitness Club" class for 30 consecutive minutes from 5 minutes. (predetermined qualitative scales of participation will be used to measure the level of participation)
- ☑ By the end of the year, student will maintain a conversation "volley" (listen/speak) for 5 minutes with a staff member on topics other than student's area of interest
- ☑ By the end of the year, student will maintain an appropriate distance from the person with whom she is speaking, without the use of prompts.
- ☑ By the end of the year, student will greet (Saying "Good morning") staff at the school office upon arrival without prompts from staff 4 out of 5 days.

- ☑ By the end of June, student will improve his use of specific social cues in a conversation or group setting by tracking his own social cues (eye contact, leaning toward speaker, nodding head) in videotapes of interactions.
- ☑ At least once a day, with gestural prompts from staff, student will use augmentative communication to interact with peers in her "Girls Group" using pre-taped riddles.
- ☑ During choral reading with the class, with gestural prompts from staff, student will use augmentative communication to repeat repetitive lines in a story book such as Brown Bear, Brown Bear.
- ☑ During group discussions, student begins to talk at the same time as another person, he will either back down to allow the other person to talk or will invite the other student to speak after he has finished his short message. Student will maintain a check mark record of his responses over the course of the day. (Garcia Winner, 2008, p.298)

Social Communication and Language Objectives:

- ☑ Using one picture and hand-over-hand, student will give a picture to an adult when he wants something and the preferred item will be given immediately. He will independently complete request sequence without prompts for 4 of 5 opportunities when trainer is in close proximity (within 1 foot).
- ☑ Will imitate functional play action by watching the play partner, then imitating the play action within 5 seconds of the presentation. The child will correctly respond in the first trial of each action with at least 4 toys across 4 consecutive days.
- ☑ During group discussions, student begins to talk at the same time as another person, he will notice the other person is talking and silence himself. A score of 3 or more will be attained on the attached rubric. (Garcia Winner, 2008, p.298)
- ☑ By the end of the semester using a pre - taught graphic organizer and script the student will write a topic sentence and three supporting details independently.
- ☑ Using a visual organizer with category images, student will correctly categorize 12 common nouns into 4 categories on at least 3 occasions by the end of the term.
- ☑ Using grade 2 stories and visual prompts, student will orally answer "wh" questions" (who, what, where) correctly 9 out of 10 times.
- ☑ During structured teaching sessions, using two communicative partners and physical prompting, items that are disliked will be offered to student and she will indicate "No" by pointing to the "No" picture card 3 out of 3 times on 5 occasions during a two week period.
- ☑ Using items known to be strongly liked as well as those strongly disliked, student will be presented with at least 5 opportunities a day to indicate personal choice by pointing to "yes" or "no" cards in natural situations.
- ☑ Using partial verbal prompts, student will match a variety of photographic food cards with the corresponding written word and name them accurately 9 out of 10 times, at least three times over a two week period.
- ☑ Using a verbal and a partial physical prompt "Do this," student will mirror the *actions of others involving body movements.* He will perform the imitation response 8 out of 10 times during natural play.

- ☑ Using a verbal and physical prompt, "Do this" student will mirror the actions of others involving the *manipulation of physical objects.* He will perform the imitation response 8 out of 10 times at his work table.
- ☑ Participate with a partner in a turn taking game for 15 minutes a day for 10 days, gradually decreasing the prompts that remind him to wait his turn, from verbal to gestural to no prompts.
- ☑ Follow teacher's 3 step instructions (visually and verbally presented) in the regular physical education class for 7 minutes daily.
- ☑ Eat lunch with a partner for 1 day in the week (parallel interaction).
- ☑ Eat lunch with a partner for 2 days a week and exchange one question/answers (prepared beforehand) to your partner.
- ☑ Eat lunch with a partner for 2 days a week and exchange 3 question/answers (prepared beforehand) to your partner.
- ☑ Daily, for one month, student will use a strategy sheet and videotaped sessions of himself in a social context to self -monitor and record the number of times he looks into the eyes of the person speaking, shows interest by leaning into the group and shows interest by either nodding or shaking his head. The number of checks will increase by 50% from the baseline data in the one month period.
- ☑ The student will list 3 ways he makes an impression, explaining what each means with 90% accuracy.
- ☑ Maintaining a perspective journal where the student records 3 good and 3 bad impressions he made about himself or someone else during the week. Student's responses will match teacher responses with 90% consistency.
- ☑ While viewing a video of a conversational group, the student will be able to accurately "guess" the emotional state of the different members over the course of the video with 75% accuracy.

<u>Self- Regulation and Emotional Development Goals</u>

- ☑ With decreasing levels of prompts by adult, the student will begin an unpreferred work task within 2 minutes, with only visual instructions of task on his desk.
- ☑ By the end of the school year, the student will increase his time on task during an unpreferred activity from 3 minutes to 20 minute periods before he uses his break card.
- ☑ By creating and utilizing a 5 Point Stress Scale with a staff member, student will improve his ability to accurately identify things that cause him stress, what it looks like, and what it feels like in his body. He will refer to the scale in order to communicate how he is feeling for 90% of the opportunities provided over the course of the school year.
- ☑ By the end of the winter, with prompting from staff the student will wear a coat outside every time he goes outside.
- ☑ Using a visual sequence strip, student will independently stand in line, order food and pay for food at the cafeteria by the end of the year.
- ☑ By June, the student will correctly identify the emotional state of people that are videotaped in a variety of settings, using context cues and nonverbal language cues. (8 out of 10 times)

- ☑ Given concrete and direct training, visual supports and fading prompts, student will correctly label flexible and stuck behaviours in himself.
- ☑ During undesirable activities or situations, student will request a break using a break card without staff prompting when needed 80% of the time. Given training, practice, visual supports and fading adult cues, student will identify and use a coping strategy from his emotional toolbox when he indicates he is stuck or upset.

Self -Regulation and Emotional Development Skills Objectives

- ☑ With physical prompts from staff, student will choose a relaxation technique such as a personal relaxation booklet or a sensory tool from a choice board to calm himself during times of anxiety and frustration and use it for 1 minute without staff intervention.
- ☑ With physical prompts from staff, student will choose a relaxation technique such as a personal relaxation booklet or a sensory tool from a choice board to calm himself during times of anxiety and frustration and use it for 3 minutes without staff intervention.
- ☑ With gestural prompts from staff, student will choose a relaxation technique such as a personal relaxation booklet or a sensory tool from a choice board to calm himself during times of anxiety and frustration and use it for 1 minute without staff intervention.
- ☑ Given his 5 point stress scale and a matching data sheet, student will check in 3 times daily with a staff member to practice rating his stress level and note it on his data sheet throughout the month of October. (It would be optimal if student's 5 Point stress scale would be reviewed at <u>home</u> and with <u>other teachers</u> (at least 2) that work with student and utilized consistently.
- ☑ Using a reinforcement system, student will increase his use of a break card to request a break before reaching a level 4 on the 5 point Scale for 50% of opportunities over a two week period (gradually increase to 90% over time).
- ☑ Using a reinforcement system, the student will express her feelings by placing an arrow on an emotion scale to communicate to staff how she is feeling. Staff will prompt after waiting 30 seconds for the student to complete the skill.
- ☑ Student will begin a task within 15 seconds with 4 verbal reminders by staff by December. (Fade verbal prompts and shorten time span in each objective. Reinforce the appropriate action.)
- ☑ Using a visual sequence strip with script, student will wait quietly in line behind one other person to order food in the cafeteria (no yelling out). The number of people in front of him will gradually increase over time)
- ☑ Using a prompter, to physically prompt (partial), student will hand a break card to the communicative partner during work tasks at his desk 90% of the time. A timer will indicate the end of the two minute break. Student will return to the task 100% of the time.
- ☑ A prompter will gestually and/or visually prompt student to hand a break card to the communicative partner during times of rising frustration (80% of the time). Student will return to the task 100% of the time after break has been taken.

- ☑ Following direct teaching of how to keep an anger record, the student will use the "Daily Anger Record" (taken from Preparing for Life, Jed Baker) each time he experiences anger for one week. The student will fill out the first half describing what upset him and then complete the second half about how he handled the situation. This will be done independently only after the skill has been successfully mastered with the guidance of staff.

Cognitive and Executive Functioning Goals

- ☑ By the end of the year, student will use a graphic story plan organizer to create a short story independently.
- ☑ By the end of the school year, student will independently create a visual list of required materials to complete an assignment, pack the materials in her schoolbag and bring them to class.
- ☑ By the end of the school year, student will reduce the impulse to interrupt activities (3 days with no interruptions) inappropriately, using the visual cues on his desk without prompts from staff.
- ☑ By the end of the semester, given a home-school homework checklist and an auditory reminder (alarm on his phone), student will complete and hand in homework and assignments across all academic subjects, 90% of opportunities, given direct verbal cues to use his checklist and reinforcement for doing so.
- ☑ By the end of the year, student will sequence a 5 step picture sequence 9 out of 10 times with no prompts from staff.
- ☑ By June, the student will use picture and context cues to make one reasonable prediction about a story plot that is written at his reading comprehension level.

Cognitive and Executive Functioning Objectives

- ☑ Student will choose one from 3 possible options (written), the most appropriate prediction of a character's emotions in a story that is read to him. He will accurately identify the emotion 3 out of 5 times.
- ☑ Student will choose one from 6 possible options (written), the most appropriate prediction of a character's emotions in a story that is read to him. He will accurately identify the emotion 3 out of 5 times.
- ☑ By the end of 2 weeks the student will complete one step in a 3 step instruction, physically remove the picture symbol that represents that step and put it in an "All Done," folder with a verbal and gestural prompt from staff.
- ☑ By the end of 4 weeks the student will complete each step in a 3 step instruction, physically remove the picture symbol that represents each step and put it in an "All Done," folder with only a gestural prompt from staff.
- ☑ Student will brainstorm and record 3 possible reasons why he should have time to play with a toy (preferred activity) based on guiding questions from staff.
- ☑ Student will brainstorm and record 5 possible reasons why he should have time to play with a toy (preferred activity) without any prompts or questions from staff.
- ☑ In order to develop note taking skills later, the student will listen to 5 sentences and correctly identify 5 key words in sentences. By the end of the semester student will be able to identify key words in a sentence 80% of the time.

Academic Goals

- ☑ By the end of the year, student will accurately identify the names of coins and bills (penny, nickel, dime, quarter and bills up to fifty dollars) 9 out of 10 times.
- ☑ By the end of the year, student will accurately identify the values of a penny, nickel, dime, quarter and bills up to fifty dollars with 90% accuracy.
- ☑ By the end of the year, student will use money functionally by counting out the correct amount asked for, 8 out of 10 times.
- ☑ In a classroom setting, when given a three digit number student will count up by 5's with 9 out of 10 correct responses in 3 out of 4 consecutive trials.
- ☑ By the end of the year, student will read the thermometer accurately 90% of the time when asked.
- ☑ When presented with fractional models of halves, fourths, thirds, sixths and eighths in with mixed numerators, student will correctly name the fractional parts in 8 out of 10 opportunities as observed by a teacher at three different probes.
- ☑ By the end of the year, student will match 50 vocabulary words to pictures accurately 80% of the time.
- ☑ By the end of the year, student will demonstrate improved reading comprehension by using picture symbols to respond to questions about a text with pictures. Accuracy will be 80%.
- ☑ Student will match the number of objects in a set with the correct numeral and number word 8 out of 10 times.

Academic Skill Objectives

- ☑ Student will demonstrate comprehension of a short text by answering yes/no questions accurately (using index cards) 4 out of 5 times by the end of the semester.
- ☑ Student will add two one digit numbers accurately 8 out of 10 times with the support of concrete manipulatives but not a calculator.
- ☑ Student will accurately identify the values of a penny, nickel, dime and quarter with 90% accuracy by matching money values visually.
- ☑ Student will pair words to symbols to accurately identify and name the signs and symbols of math (+, -, =, $) by the end of the semester.
- ☑ The student will correctly identify the appropriate comparative word (provided on cue cards) to describe two objects (big, small) 5 out of 8 times.
- ☑ Using a visual checklist of steps, student will subtract two digit numbers with regrouping using a place value mat, with 80% accuracy by the end of the month.
- ☑ With partial physical prompts, student will match a sentence with the corresponding picture 8 out of 10 times correctly.
- ☑ With physical prompts, student will use a ruler to measure 5 objects accurately for five consecutive trials.
- ☑ With only partial prompts, student will put 5 events from a familiar story in proper sequence 8 out of 10 times.
- ☑ Will complete a non-preferred close ended math task, while staying seated in small group for 10 minutes in 50% of opportunities for 4 consecutive days.

Self Help and Daily Living Goals

The purpose of self- help and daily living skills is always to improve daily living skills and to increase personal abilities for greater independence. This is prudent planning for future transition out of high school. It is also wise to incorporate sexuality training for older students.

- ☑ By the end of the year, the student will put on "pull-up" (pants with elastic waistbands, underpants, or tights garments) correctly without assistance 8 out of 10 times over a two week period.
- ☑ By June, student will independently complete each step of washing his hands using only a visual schedule.
- ☑ By June, using a visual checklist, student will independently complete washing, drying and folding a basket of laundry over 5 different probes in one month.
- ☑ By the end of the year, the student will identify his address (in verbal or non – verbal means) when asked by a person outside of the classroom 8 out of 10 times correctly.
- ☑ Student will put shoes on correct feet without assistance 9 out of 10 times by June.
- ☑ By the end of the school year, student will complete the steps of a visual recipe independently to cook a desired food item.
- ☑ By June, the student will follow the visual steps outlined to launder her clothes independently, in the washing machine.
- ☑ After gym class, using a visual checklist, student will remove his clothes from the locker and dress himself independently 3 out of 3 opportunities for 4 consecutive weeks.

Self Help and Daily Living Objectives

- ☑ Practicing once a week for two months, the student will gather all of the ingredients for making a sandwich by reading a visual recipe card and verbal prompts from staff. The student will complete each step with the aid of the visual cue and verbal prompts from staff.
- ☑ Practicing once a week for a month, the student will gather all of the ingredients for making a sandwich by reading a visual recipe card. The student will complete each step with the aid of the visual cue. (No prompts from staff.)
- ☑ Student will correctly match the temperature on the thermometer with the appropriate clothing in a matching activity 6 out of 8 times with no prompts by the end of the semester.
- ☑ After gym class, using a visual checklist and verbal prompts, student will remove his clothes from the locker and dress himself 3 out of 3 opportunities for 2 consecutive weeks.

Teaching Strategies

The following list of strategies is the main topic of my second book, *One Step at a Time*. Based on scientific evidence, the following methods, although far from a comprehensive list, are an excellent fit for students with autism (and just good teaching). It is well worth the time and effort for teachers to familiarize themselves with the teaching methods associated with Applied Behaviour Analysis, as they are profoundly effective in a regular classroom (not to be confused with clinical procedures).

- Task analysis
- Discrete-trial training
- Pivotal response training
- Prompting
- Fading
- Shaping
- Modeling
- Forward Chaining/Backward Chaining
- Functional Behavioural Assessment
- Video modeling
- Social Scripting/Script Fading
- Structured peer-play interactions
- Incidental teaching
- Generalization
- Data collection
- Reinforcement

Assessment Methods

- Demonstration of the skill
- Success Criteria
- Checklist
- Data Collection
- Written Activity (using pen and paper or the computer)
- Oral Response
- Matching Exercise
- Cloze Procedure
- Qualitative Scale
- Sorting Exercises

Linking the IEP to the Report Card

Throughout the term, teachers are expected to monitor a student's progress towards the goals and objectives on the IEP. This would be one reason that storing the IEP in a drawer is not productive! Progress is summarized on the Report Card. The fact that a student has an IEP will have to be indicated on the report card. This is usually not the case for IEPs that consist of accommodations only. If only accommodations have been made, the evaluative statement reflects the grade level curricular outcomes. On the other hand, progress in modified **and/or** alternative programs goals will be directly reported on the report card.

The Report Card is directly linked to the IEP because it reports on the student's progress towards the goals and objectives stated in the IEP.

What if This Was Your Child?

Report card time delivers a nasty sting for parents of children with autism. Fourteen years after a diagnosis and I still cringe when I read our son's report from the school. I would ask administration and educators to read the report with the eyes and the heart of a parent or loved one because only then would we see that our choice of words can be disheartening and downright exasperating.

I am not suggesting that we should "flower" a report so that it feels good for a parent or a child. To do so would be equally inappropriate. Think of Goldilocks. The bed that she liked the best at the Three Bears' house was not too soft and not too hard. Report cards need to be realistic, not mean. They must report on the IEP goals and progress towards regular curriculum, if appropriate.

In our haste to complete these time sucking documents we might overlook the devastating impact our words can have. Below Standard. Failing to improve. Needs to work harder. Are we too focused on deficits? Report cards often make value judgments on a skill that is an area of deficit because the child is autistic: fine motor, self -control, organization, initiation and such are often assessed as below average. What is the point of stating that little Beth is not meeting the standard for working in a group? She has autism – of course she is below the standard! If she needs improvement then we, the educators, must ask ourselves if we are working to build that skill on the IEP! **Unless the school team is doing something to teach these areas (and the goals are in the IEP) they should never show up on a report card!**

"Catching up" isn't the goal for our kids with autism. Learners are not all on the same path- despite what standardized tests and curriculum say. Making progress towards meaningful individual goals is the reason we send our kids to school isn't it? A student may be far from the state or provincial standard but a report card should report the progress the child has made in a goal. One parent reported to me that her son's report was based on the average child so despite making huge progress it appeared that he hadn't achieved much at all. Nowhere did it mention that in six months he'd gone from not writing to writing whole stories.

Report cards need to be meaningful and authentic. A student's areas of growth must balance the areas that still need work. There is absolutely no place for demeaning comments based on assumptions. After all, what may look like disruptive behaviour is very likely neurologically based. In addition, the behaviour points to what we as professionals need to be doing to address the message that is being communicated. I remember so well that whenever our son seemed to be "regressing" or failing to progress the team in charge of his programming would always reflect on what needed to be changed in the program NOT how our son needed to change. That lesson has stayed with me. **What do we need to change so that the child makes progress?**

At the same time, report cards that are overly "fluffy" and filled with glowing remarks are equally inappropriate. Report cards will be used in decision making for future planning for a child with autism. Transitions to post- secondary schooling and adult life will necessitate a review of the student's academic life, strengths and needs. They must be authentic reflections of the individual. Teachers who do not want to hurt or demoralize a parent or child must do so by balancing the comments about growth and areas of continued need for support. This is not the place to gloss over the needs of a student.

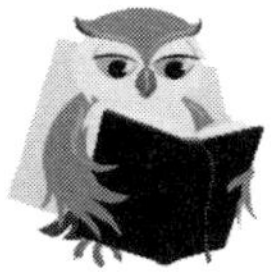

If a child can't learn the way we teach, maybe we should teach the way they learn.

-Ignacio 'Nacho' Estrada

Taming Transitions

Ah, the dreaded transition or change in routine! Just mention to the teacher or parent of an autistic child that some plan has changed and you will witness a subtle twitch and a tremble! Transitions are very difficult for students with autism and so it is imperative that we provide supports that help students to cope. Rather than trying to "move mountains" to avoid changes, let's give the student the tools he needs to deal with the stress of change. Life is full of change and the better the child will be if we do the groundwork. By building a toolbox and facilitating its consistent use, our children can avoid being "swallowed up in anxiety."

Each provincial Ministry of Education in Canada and the U.S. Department of Education make it very clear that planning for transitions is an integral part of a student's individual education plan. Planning for transitions, even minor ones, needs to be well thought out and systematically implemented. Students should have formal transition plans in place at least by the time they are in junior high school (aged 13 or 14). But, students with autism need a plan in place throughout the school years.

Transition into the school system

- Plan school/classroom visits well in advance of actual start date. It may take several short visits with gradually increasing lengths of time for the student to adjust and feel more comfortable
- Review a video of the school many times with prospective student (introducing the classroom, gymnasium, hallways, and all relevant people including the principal, secretary, and custodial staff)
- An introductory video describing school rules and procedures (including uniforms, clubs, homework and attendance policies) will show expectations visually
- Use children's story books about going to school and create a personal story about the child going to school (use real pictures of the school in Clicker 5, Powerpoint or movie maker)

Transition between grade levels

- Meet with the teacher to discuss the child's needs, strengths (Use the Portrait of a Student template as a place to begin)
- Classroom visits by receiving teacher
- A Social Story™ book (Carol Gray) should be developed and sent home
- Examine and consider materials and strategies that are being used successfully and those that have not been productive
- When entering high school the same effective strategies should be employed as were when the child entered school
- An older student (a compassionate and reliable one) could have his locker next to the student with autism so that he can monitor transition times and come to the aid of the student if something is not right
- Locks with only one number combination are available...the student should be practicing opening the lock before school starts

- Color coded binders that match a color coded timetable support executive function
- Invite next year's student to have lunch with you at school (this is a big hit with parents, teachers and kids!)

Transition between activities and settings
- Show the child that you are changing the visual schedule
- Use visual clocks, timers, warnings and ample time – avoid overly verbal explanations and warnings
- Use First /Then schedules, first/next/then visual schedules
- Use peer buddies to facilitate movement
- Implement early or late release times
- Use a transition object - use an object to indicate what is coming next (lunch bag means lunch, calculator means math, ball means gym etc…)
- Use a favourite object to motivate transition (teddy bear goes to circle time)

Transitions from Secondary School to Adult Life
A formal Transition Plan is part of the Individual Education Plan by law at 14 years of age. A transition plan is a detailed document highlighting the future needs of an individual and how these needs will be met. It addresses core areas such as further education, health, housing, transportation, work, relationships and hobbies.

Life Transitions in General
- Draw comic pictures and write brief stories describing the new situation
- Prepare a directory of the new staff members or key people's names
- Prepare a floor plan, map or video of a new place
- Create a list of towns that will be passed on route to a destination
- Use a calendar to indicate the important dates, times etc…
- Teach the skills needed to say goodbye, stay in contact with old friends and manage anxiety
- Use a Power Card strategy to reinforce that favorite characters accept change, and cope positively with different situations (divorce, death, remarriage, moving, etc…)
- Use a transition object that the student always carries in transitions

3) Integrating a Transition Plan

The very nature of autism complicates the transition of a student from high school into the adult world. The challenges around communication, sensory regulation, behaviour, cognitive differences and the social impairments can complicate transition planning. Schools, students and parents need to work together to be proactive in their planning. But, it takes a community to welcome these individuals into society as a whole.

Students should be as autonomous as possible in the decisions that impact the future. To the degree possible, and with the guidance and support of the school and home, a student with autism should be involved in identifying their interests, experimenting with different work placements and choosing living arrangements. With the help of school staff, parents and community liaisons students have to be prepared and made aware of the options they are facing. Students need to understand the changes that are happening to the extent possible. This is more complex for a student with autism and the information needs to be presented in a way that is meaningful and minimally anxiety provoking – usually visually and concretely.

The school, in collaboration with the parents, will need to educate potential employers, job coaches and community agencies about the areas of need in which the student may need accommodations or at minimum, greater understanding:

- Communication and language
- Social interactions
- Sensory and perceptual challenges
- Cognitive patterns (the need for routine and predictable environments, executive function problems, difficulties with flexible thinking)

By 14 years of age and older, students need to have a formal Transition Plan that is aimed at putting in place the student's course of study (advanced placement and courses or vocational study programs). A transition plan must also serve the purpose of preparing the student to make the transition from the world of the school to the "real" world and adulthood. This plan is critical in outlining any interagency involvement from the community. The transition plan must include appropriate**, measurable** post-secondary goals that are based on the **individual student's needs** and that take into account the student's **strengths, preferences, and interests**. The plan must also be updated annually.

To be meaningful and useful, the transition services (the document plus the courses and activities) must be **results oriented** and directly related to helping students improve their academic and functional achievement so that they can successfully move to:

- College/University
- Vocational training and apprenticeship programs
- Supported employment – educators look for employers who hire students with special needs and a job coach or supervisor oversees the student
- Independent living

As if surviving the early years of raising a child with autism isn't enough, parents need to be thinking practically about the future of a child from the beginning. It can be painful to think that far ahead. To be clear, I am not speaking of the anxiety laden, fretful kind of 'thinking ahead.' More constructive, is the kind of thinking that leads to leaving doors open for your child. For example, when you and your child's educational team are developing an IEP in elementary school, keep in mind that the decisions you make in this IEP could affect the child's opportunities later. If your child is participating in the grade level regular curriculum and the standardized testing of the state or province, the door remains open to earning credits to obtain a high school diploma. Even if a child will not likely live independently, there are still many skills which need to be taught to ensure an autonomous and content life.

"Time flies." This fact is especially true for parents of special needs children. Days turn into months and months into years and while we are busy with the day to day challenges of raising a child with autism, time has brought our child to high school.

Transition planning requires a lot of inter-agency discussion and work. This is often a challenging task because each agency has a mandate, limited resources and an agenda. From the start, each person or agencies roles and responsibilities need to be clear. The involvement of a number of agencies requires that communication is a priority and all persons involved in the process will need a sound understanding and awareness of the unique needs of individuals living with autism. I know this sounds like a tall order – it is. Ultimately, we can only be responsible for *our* own words, actions and attitudes, not anyone else's.

> "All aspects of individual's life need to be taken into consideration within the transition *plan to ensure they are given options that reflect their desired future direction. The transition plan should address core areas such as further education, health, housing, transport, work, relationships and hobbies. With all areas it is important that the individual understands what each route involves and how it will affect them… It is important that visits are made to all prospective providers and/or further education establishments allowing the individual to make an informed decision. The following are some factors to consider: location, size of the place, number of staff, level of support offered, environmental issues (noise), ASD training and experience."*
>
> The National Autistic Society, www.nas.org.uk

Dr. Jed Baker's book, entitled, *Preparing for Life,* is an excellent resource for planning the skills necessary for students with high- functioning autism. The book covers all of the deficit areas, the dire need for generalization of skills, and social skills training that these students will need in order to be successfully integrated into their community. Jed Baker correctly emphasizes that the skills he presents are meant to *augment* the unique personality of students, **not** to make them more typical and more "socially correct."

Who Should be a Part of Transition Planning?

- Student
- Parent
- Special education teacher or related services provider
- Regular education teacher
- Guidance counselors
- Vocational educators
- Administrators
- Local agencies, workplace representatives, job coaches, related service providers

What Information is Needed?

When planning the transition from high school to the adult world of post - secondary and workplace settings there are specific pieces of information that are needed to make meaningful and relevant decisions:

- ✓ Knowledge of the student's out of school activities, hobbies, career interests and needs – based on parent and student surveys, interest inventories and functional vocational assessments
- ✓ The student's Individual Education Plan and school records that are relevant to future functioning of the student (report cards and educational assessments, out of school professional assessments)
- ✓ A list of potential local agencies and contact persons
- ✓ School board policies and possible school board agreements with educational providers and institutions, local employers, local service providers
- ✓ Health services that the student is currently receiving
- ✓ Social skills assessments (as noted by Jed Baker in the book, *Preparing for Life*, Future Horizons Inc.)

It is beneficial for a student (staff or parent) keep a portfolio of documents that will be relevant to the transition process as the teenage years unfold.

Transition Activities:

For students with autism, skill development should never be left to chance. Explicit instruction in the academic, vocational, and adult living skills is needed to achieve transition goals. I am a firm believer in the necessity of specific and explicit teaching of self-advocacy and self-awareness for kids on the spectrum. In order to be autonomous, students need to be aware of their disability and how it impacts their lives and their thinking. For example, a student with autism should realize that at times, he perseverates on his favorite topic. He may ask a peer, teacher or job coach to give a predetermined signal that he is "doing it again" if he doesn't catch this habit himself. Our son has been taught to be aware of areas of weakness (organizing and planning) so that he is willing and able to seek support and use the compensatory tools he has been taught.

- ✓ Conduct assessments of student needs, interests or preferences for future education, employment, and adult living – examine recreation and leisure activities
- ✓ Determine which curricular expectations need to be integrated into the individual education plan to meet the transition goals
- ✓ Provide opportunities for student to try out various workplace placements that match his or her interests

- ✓ Visit potential post -secondary institutions; discuss the policies and systems for support of individuals with autism (address how the student will obtain organizational support, social supports, and academic accommodations)
- ✓ Many post -secondary institutions require a recent psycho-educational assessment in order to prove the diagnosis and to identify the accommodations and supports that will be needed
- ✓ Identify and provide the accommodations, supports, or related services that the student needs in their present education in order to meet their future transition goals
- ✓ Provide information about independent living alternatives; begin the application process
- ✓ Seek information about post school financial options and support; begin the application process
- ✓ Begin the application process for housing or begin the process of seeking appropriate housing
- ✓ Teach students and families about how students can assume the role of primary decision maker in their futures
- ✓ Identify assistive technology that can be used as the student transitions to employment or postsecondary education
- ✓ Connect with adult services organizations and help families identify resources and supports in their community – the community people need to be made aware and educated about the nature of autism – it cannot be assumed that the general public understands this complex disorder
- ✓ Provide for planning follow-up or follow-along support once the student develops independence in a transition activity or once he graduates

The scope of the skills that need to be explicitly taught and generalized for effective transition is enormous. The following is a sampling of the kinds of skills that students need to be learning during their school years:

- Self -awareness and self -advocacy
- Coping with anger/anxiety and frustration
- Non -verbal language (facial cues, gestures, body language etc…)
- Building and maintaining friendships and work relationships
- Conversation skills
- Employment skills (interview skills, searching for a job, coping with rejection, criticism and complaints, writing resumes etc…)
- Saving money, spending within one's means, banking
- Job skills (stocking shelves, sorting, stapling, using a list, delivering etc…) Personal appearance and hygiene

- Completing application forms
- Making telephone calls
- Using public transportation (using a bus schedule, calling a cab, driver's license)
- Social skills with customers
- Cleaning skills (both general and systematic)
- Washing, folding laundry
- Food purchasing and preparation
- Healthy living
- Managing pedestrian rules, traffic, traffic signs
- Using public facilities such as washrooms
- Finding and using community services such as pools, recreation centers, banks, drugstores, and grocery stores
- Using restaurant skills such as choosing, ordering food and paying
- Using postal services and email

Once a student is 14 years of age, he or she should be invited to attend the education plan/transition meeting. It is essential that by this age students begin to play a key role in their educational planning. We are all more likely to take ownership and responsibility for something that we have had a hand in developing. This is no different for teenagers. Students should know what is in their individual education plan, why it is there and how they can advocate for their needs. It is beneficial for teachers or guidance counselors to "coach" a student and explicitly teach them the skills of asking for clarification, stating strengths and needs, interests and preferences. Families also need to be actively involved. If the student does not attend, the school personnel must make sure that the student's preferences, interests and goals are represented.

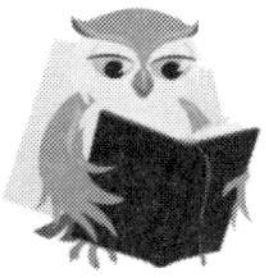

> **"On our own we simply don't know how to get things done the same way you do things. But, like everyone else, we want to do the best we possibly can. When we sense you've given up on us, it makes us feel miserable. So please keep helping us, through to the end."**
>
> **Naoki Higashida**
> ***The Reason I Jump: The Inner Voice of a Thirteen-Year-Old Boy with Autism***

IDEA 2004 Transition Checklist

The list below describes the required components of the transition plan in the United States. Although it does not describe Canadian law, the author feels that the checklists are excellent tools for parents and teachers in Canada as well as in the U. S. During a student's high school years, it is essential that the IEP team adhere to these requirements.

- ☑ The student must be invited to participate in IEP meetings to discuss his/her goals for life after high school.
- ☑ You may request several IEP/Transition Planning meetings during the school year.
- ☑ You may invite representatives of local agencies to these IEP meetings to discuss transition goals and services to support those goals.
- ☑ The IEP, including the transition plan, should be based on person-centered planning, and reflect the student's interests and skills.
- ☑ The work experiences or "community based work assessments" (CBWAs) chosen should be based on the student's interests and abilities. Students should NOT be placed in a community based work assessment simply because it is available.
- ☑ Any placement should help the student develop skills in a setting that is of personal interest to him/ her and where his/her unique abilities can be successfully utilized and improved with job coaching.
- ☑ Annual transition goals in the IEP should lead to successful post- high school outcomes.
- ☑ Progress should be documented and measurable.
- ☑ Ask for progress reports about your child's community based work experience. Discuss with the IEP team how your child will meet the goal of being employed after graduation, without a lapse in supports and services.
- ☑ Maintain a portfolio and resume of your child's experiences, progress reports, and favorable reviews from your child's supervisors.

Transition Planning Checklist

While IDEA 2004 provides the legal requirements for transition services to support your child's goal of employment in the community or further education, there are several things that parents and students must do to prepare for life after high school. The following is an excellent resource to ensure that you are on the right track in planning for your child's future. Written by Jennifer Graham and Peter Wright

Transition Task	Done
Confirm the date of your child's graduation. Federal law states that your child's eligibility for special education ends when s/he graduates from high school with a regular diploma or until the child reaches the age of eligibility for a free appropriate education under State law.	
Clarify whether your child will receive a regular high school diploma or a certificate of attendance.	
Clarify that your child will be able to fully participate in the graduation ceremony.	
Find out what local agencies provide job coaching for transitioning youth. Contacting adult provider agencies before your child graduates or "ages out" will help to ensure that your child will continue to receive services after graduation. This may also prevent your child from being placed on a long waiting list for adult services.	
You are entitled to invite representatives from other agencies to your child's IEP meetings.	
If the IEP Team, which includes the parents and the child, determine that your child's transition needs can be met by participating in transition programs on college campuses or in community based settings, these services should be included in the child's IEP.	
If appropriate, invite the child's supports coordinator from your local Office of Mental Retardation to IEP meetings during the last year of high school. This person can help to coordinate post-high school support services.	
If your child will be eligible for services through Vocational Rehabilitation, schedule an appointment for an intake interview and file the necessary paperwork with the Office of Vocational Rehabilitation ahead of time. Request that a Vocational Rehabilitation counselor attend the IEP meeting no later than spring of your child's last year in high school.	
Discuss your child's transportation needs. If s/he will need assistance getting to and from work, request and fill out applications for public transportation services.	
Request information about social/recreational opportunities for young adults with disabilities in your community. Ask for their contact information.	
Request information about post-high school training programs at local vocational schools, community colleges, business schools, and state-affiliated training schools.	

Are we There Yet?

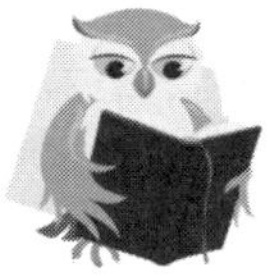

> ***Success is to be measured not so much by the position one has reached in life, as by the obstacles which one has overcome while trying to succeed.***
>
> ***Booker T. Washington***

4) Implementing the IEP: Keeping it Real

Take a deep breath. Pat yourself on the back. The document is complete. The parents have signed it. The legal expectations have been met. **JUST KIDDING.** Actually, the work has just begun! Education plans are a process, not a product. If we create them and put them away we have wasted our time. In this light, the education plans are just a bureaucratic hoop to jump through.

How do we keep individual education plans real? **Keep the document close** and record what's working and what's not working. Monitor and track a student's progress. At times when you are not directly teaching the student, ask an educational assistant or support worker to keep a notebook that provides a brief description of what worked with a student on that day in that objective. Objective data can be collected by anyone working with the student. Anyone who has worked with autistic students knows the frustration of a skill being performed one day and not the next! Anecdotal notes or tracking sheets (examples provided as templates in Appendices) help to keep a teacher informed of progress.

Don't be afraid to **write on the IEP**, put sticky notes, check marks, anything that you need to do to make it alive and dynamic! Some teachers find that within a few months into the year, the student's goals have changed and the goals and/or expectations need revision. In working with students with autism, we often discover prerequisite sub-skills that are needed before acquiring the next level of skill. For example, a student with autism may be able to identify the names of coins and the values but he may not be able to demonstrate functional use of those coins until he has mastered and generalized the skill of matching different coins with varying values (one quarter = one nickel and two dimes or five pennies and four nickels). It's not until we are in the thick of teaching that we realize what steps are missing.

One method of checking in on the status of a learning expectation is called **probing**. Periodically, a teacher should ask or prompt the student to demonstrate the skill that has been taught. Keep a record of how many times the student accurately demonstrates the skill. This is especially important once a skill has been mastered and generalized. If the student has been learning his address, it does not take much effort to have the secretary "spontaneously" ask the child for his address. The response he gives will give a good indication of whether that skill has yet been truly mastered.

Keeping an individual education plan "real" requires that the objectives and goals set out are **incorporated into the daily plan** of the student. This does not have to be a make work project for the teacher. It requires forethought, but it will go a long way towards meeting the student's needs. Examine the daily plans and schedule for the class. Notice where the objectives outlined fall into the schedule for the day and "plug them" into a personal schedule for the student. For example, if an objective is for Betty to identify the names of 3 geometric figures by the end of the month; then it is imperative that somewhere on Betty's visual schedule she have a word or a symbol for shape discrimination.

The tricky goals to monitor are the ones that require **frequent tracking**. For example, in a class of 30 students it is quite challenging for the teacher to note every time the child raises her hand before leaving the room (if that is a goal). One way that works effectively is to give the responsibility to the student for putting a "check mark" every time she raises her hand before she leaves the room. This can greatly reduce negative behaviours and increase positive ones because the student is expected to be aware of and accountable for her actions. Even young children will be able to use check marks for expected behaviours. Just remember to incorporate reinforcement for achieving objectives!

Parents of secondary students are concerned that goals and objectives become lost in the hustle of running from one class to another. This is a very valid concern and one that requires a carefully thought out plan. Again, a chart of the student's courses and a tracking sheet should be part of the student's binder. Regular classroom teachers can oversee the student's self – tracking. For less abled students, the educational assistant or teacher would need to take this responsibility.

A "**travel card**" is a useful tool that ensures that the student's objectives are being tracked in each class. A grid format can be created with a list of the objectives (academic, social, cognitive, behavioural etc...) that the student is working towards. List the student's classes on the one side or axis and the objectives on the other. The objectives MUST be observable and measurable so that the teacher in each class can quickly check which objectives were met that day. The teacher initials the card and the student proceeds to his next class. The student would receive a personally motivating form of reinforcement for carrying the card as well as engaging in the targeted objectives or behaviours.

The following is a very informal idea of what a task card might look like. Teachers or students would check off which objectives were met and make comments if necessary. Each travel card could be designed for one particular class and color coded to match the text and the timetable. Travel cards could also outline the objectives for all classes.

Objective	Monday	Tuesday	Wednesday	Thursday	Friday
Write 3 sentences in journal.					
Bring text, notebook, pencil and calculator.					
Identify a square, circle and triangle.					
Record names of characters on a story web.					

OR the following demonstrates a more appropriate travel card for social and self-management objectives.

Objective	Math	English	Science	Music	History
Stay in seat for 10 minute intervals.					
Bring text, notebook, pencil and necessary tools					
Raise hand before responding to a general question.					
Ask one question during group work.					
Use a break card instead of leaving class without permission.					

It is not the sole responsibility of a special education teacher to teach the skills that a student with autism needs to learn. All educators share the responsibility and all educators must use the IEP as a meaningful document. It is easy for some teachers to "slough" off the IEP as "just a student's crutch," or "someone else's job." But, in the end, each teacher would be well served by asking themselves how they would want their own child or nephew treated if he had autism. We have an ethical duty to teach each and every child - not just the ones that are easy to teach. The IEP is an efficient way to do just that.

Communication with parents is another key to keeping the plan real and effective. When parents are well informed of what is going on in the educational plans they can (and should) work on those same skills at home. This improves the chances of generalizing the skill (having the child demonstrate it in more than one place, at different times and with different people) significantly. Just a short note, email or a telephone call to say that one of the goals or expectations needs to be "tweaked" because the child needs to learn a sub skill first is a good way to keep parents informed and feeling like they are a part of a team. Parents may also want to share an idea with the teacher without going through a formal team meeting.

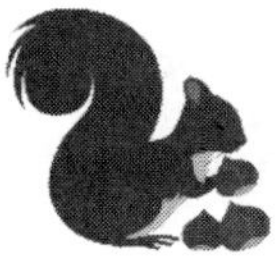

Keeping it Real, in a Nutshell:

- ✓ Keep the document in close proximity (or at least a working version of it)
- ✓ Take data to Monitor and track a student's progress
- ✓ Write on the IEP
- ✓ Probe for skill retention regularly
- ✓ Incorporate objectives into the daily plan of the student
- ✓ Implement self- tracking and delegate data collection
- ✓ Ensure ALL educators share responsibility
- ✓ Keep communication open and frequent between home and school

5) Are We There Yet? Assessment Drives Instruction

Once during every reporting period the education plan must be formally reviewed and updated. Teachers assess the student's acquisition of the skills either using formal or informal assessments. At this point teachers need to examine the data collected, the anecdotal records, the checklists and the observation sheets that were used when a student was learning the skill. Based on the assessment, professional judgment will determine whether the instruction has been effective. If the student is not making progress in achieving the goals and objectives, then the teacher needs to change the instructional methods or resources. Assessment must directly impact instructional decisions. We have to meet the child where the child is at in the here and now. We can't possibly try to make the student fit the instruction!

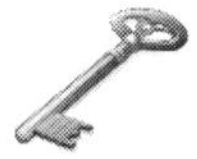

The Key to Success: Communication

Research shows that the most effective way to build positive relationships is to keep the lines of communication open at all times. The more communication that happens between a teacher and a parent the more a mutual rapport will develop. While I am not so naïve to think that this is always the case, I do believe that parents just want to be involved and to know what is happening. When they are left out, distrust and resentment begin to build. This is *their* child; they have a right and a responsibility to be a part of the child's school life.

Parents of typical students often complain that their children tell them nothing about what is going on a t school. Students with autism, even the high functioning students, are often unable to articulate or narrate the events that occurred. Teachers of non - verbal students MUST write a note home or keep a home school communication log daily because otherwise the parents have NO idea what transpired during the day with their child. Imagine if you had no clue what your child's life was like for six hours a day –

especially if your child was vulnerable. The note doesn't have to share anything earth shattering but it sure is a good start to positive rapport. Students who are capable of keeping a daily log in a book or on the computer can be responsible for the daily communication. The teacher only needs to add anything that he or she feels is important to share if there is something.

It was the end of the year before I ever knew that our son had been a part of a school drama club for the whole year! Despite being 11 years old with high functioning autism, our son countered our questioning with the fact that we had never asked that specific question! Not surprisingly, he had never brought home any of the notes that the teacher sent. Most parents and teachers would agree that our students should not be the liaison between home and school!

The following are a few ideas for notes home. Tell about:

- ☺ two activities that the child participated in
- ☺ two activities that the student enjoyed or not
- ☺ something new that the student tried
- ☺ a person that the student played with
- ☺ something that you are excited about
- ☺ something that students need to bring to school (money, a T shirt, art supplies)
- ☺ a sensory issue that arose
- ☺ a behaviour that occurred (or not!)
- ☺ a skill that was acquired
- ☺ progress that was noted

The Role of Parents

Communicate. Communicate. Communicate. Leaving communication up to the teacher is counterproductive. Waiting for the teacher to call is a waste of time and it is a sure way to build resentment. The more information you share in the form of emails, phone calls, notes and meetings the better prepared your child's teacher will be to plan appropriate strategies and set up the environment to meet your child's needs.

It is not in your child's best interest to hide or keep medical information, portions of professional assessments (especially the parts that pertain to educational recommendations) or other relevant information from your child's teacher. Students lose when parents and teachers fail to have a respectful relationship with each other. They become the victims of resentment and pride. Even the most severely challenged students with autism can "sense" strife in the relationship between parent and teacher, just as they can sense tension between their parents.

Read the teacher's notes and newsletters. As a teacher I know firsthand that my attempts at communication are often left in a crumpled pile at the bottom of the student's backpack! Okay, I must admit that I too, am guilty of not going through my children's school bags at times! But if someone takes the time to communicate with you, it sends a negative message whether intended or not.

Take every opportunity to share with the teacher what you know about your child. Avoid leaving important things about your child for the teacher to figure out, as teachers have many children under their care. This is wasted time for your child. Parents are the experts on details about their child. Parents know what transitions are difficult, what motivates the child (what reinforcers are valued), what overwhelms the child and what strategies and techniques have been the most effective/least effective.

At the same time, respect the professionalism of the teacher you are working with. You may be the expert on some aspects of your child, but teachers have extensive training in education that other professionals do not. Teachers are experts on teaching groups of children. They are well educated in the art of educating many children at one time. Over decades of teaching I have met parents that think that because they *attended* school, they know what they need to know about education.

Parent sometimes complain that their child's teacher doesn't want the parents in the classroom. Perhaps they are hiding something? Would you feel unnerved if your child's teacher were to come into your home to 'help' or to 'observe?' It is unlikely that your child would act the same way around the teacher during the visit. The same is true when you are in your child's classroom.

It also stand to reason that none of us appreciate being judged, especially when we are trying our best as a parent or a teacher. If we welcomed into a classroom to help, then we need to be positive, optimistic and empathetic. Most of all, we need to be respectful both in and outside of the class. The saying, "walk a day in my shoes," is absolutely fundamental in the relationship between a parent and a teacher.

Make it a point to know what your child is working on in each subject. Although this is the responsibility of both parents and teachers, it is not fair to wait for the teacher to tell you what is going on with your child. Parents need to be proactive; read the child's notebooks and textbooks, ask your child to tell you one thing that they learned on that day. Don't expect anything to come from the question, "What did you learn today?" The answer will invariably be, "Nothing."

The point is that the best thing that parents can do to facilitate their child's education is to be involved, communicate often and be positive about the school system. Students instinctively know their parents feelings towards the school and an attitude of resentment, distrust and frustration will certainly affect the way your child feels about school and his teachers. If the system needs changing (and all systems consisting of humans need change and improvement) then work with it, choose to see the challenges as an optimist. Be a part of the solution and not part of the problem. Change does not happen overnight. Think about how far special education has come; we are thankfully a long ways from calling students stupid, making them wear dunce caps and hitting them for wrong answers.

Last, but certainly not least in the role of parents, is the fact that parents of children with autism need to take care of themselves. We need to put our own physical, emotional and spiritual health as a priority. I have been there. I know that we cannot give what we don't have and our kids need a lot! Linking up with support groups, respite services and staying socially connected are the keys to self -preservation. Taking time to do things we enjoy and making sure that we maintain physical health may be difficult but it is critical for our children. We instinctively "dive" into the world of autism and our whole existence can become consumed by it. This should only be a temporary state of being because we will most certainly become cynical and burned out if we do not find a balance. Our other children, our marriages and our extended family deserve our attention and energy. Shutting ourselves off from these people or taking on autism alone leaves us alone, exhausted and depleted. This can never help our children with autism.

So how do we find time to take care of everything? Start by accepting help from those who offer. There are no hero awards by doing it on our own. Seek respite support, contact high school guidance counselors and principals for recommendations of dependable students that may want community service hours or part time jobs. Join a health club with daycare service. Enroll children in activities that are good for their own development.

Research what government funding or community programs may be available and make use of them! Remembering back, my husband and I had initially decided that we didn't need to access any government money that was offered for respite services. We believed that we needed more time with our son instead of having him with a stranger while we did something else. We would have felt guilty for taking time away from him (guilt and parenting go hand in hand as you know!). Fortunately, we had a case worker that corrected our faulty, guilt ridden thinking! She made us understand that we were not "dumping" him but that we were creating opportunities for him while we regrouped and maintained our own mental health! With the help of our local high school administration and with government respite money we were able to hire students that took our son hiking, swimming, taught him how to play ball, and how to make movies. We tried to hire boys because, at the time, all of his therapists and teachers were female and we wanted a male role model (other than his dad) to socialize him. Some of these hired workers ended up volunteering to spend time with him.

We now believe that rather than being selfish, taking time for ourselves provided an awesome opportunity for our son to learn new skills, practice social skills and play skills in real life situations and most importantly, develop a sense of self -esteem! It takes time and some effort to develop leisure activities for your child and yourselves but the benefits far outweigh the cost!

Taking time for ourselves provided an awesome opportunity for our son to learn new skills, practice social skills and play skills in real life situations and most importantly, develop a sense of self -esteem!

CAUTION **Choose Your Advocates Wisely**

Special education meetings are challenging to navigate. My own husband has complained that the discussions seemed "jargony" and "over his head." This is unfortunate because parents are key members of an educational team and they deserve to be a participating member who can understand what is being said. Some parents feel more comfortable attending school meetings with an advocate. Many advocates play an effective role in asking questions, making suggestions, and clarifying points for parents.

However, advocates can have their own agendas and they can be detrimental to the collaboration efforts of a school team. It has been my experience to see advocates that alienated school staff, pushed parents into unwanted and unwarranted legal action and pitted one parent against the other. Parents have paid the price in broken marriages and the financial burden of court costs. No person should ever be expected to endure verbal abuse, including school staff! Bringing an advocate that is simply an advocate because they have a "bully mentality" or a big mouth is counterproductive for collaboration and team work. Advocates can raise tensions and make accusations that only serve to close meetings and put the child's needs on hold.

Unfortunately, some parents are misled to believe that the advocate that they hired is qualified to act as an expert in the field of autism, special education or education in general. If the need arises for outside help, I strongly urge parents to do their homework: research the people you are hiring; know their qualifications, expect nothing less than specialized knowledge and qualifications in autism (a friend who has a child with autism is not the best choice). Demand that your child's advocate will participate with integrity and character in order to build relationships that will serve your child for the long run. There are many wonderful people who have the credentials and wisdom needed to effectively advocate for children. Settle for nothing less.

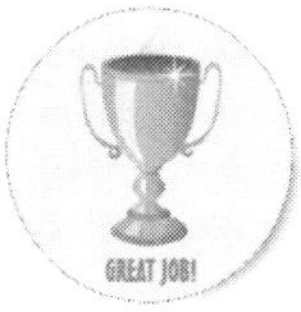

The Gold Standard: What are we Working Towards?

The educational plan is a tool. Just like any tool, it is only effective if it is used the way it was intended. Autism presents educators, parents and society with a challenge that is sure to change the face of community services, education and the workplace. Autism diagnoses are on the rise and we as a society cannot deny these individuals a life worth living. Starting with the family and the school, we need to identify and augment strengths, work to improve deficits and help each individual with autism grow into a person that values themselves and knows that they too, have a valued place in society. Increased independence is the goal; when we assume that a person can't do something and we rush in to "help" we are only enabling the disability. The people who work with autistic individuals owe it to those individuals to set up supports that empower rather than foster dependence. When we do something for someone that they could learn to do for themselves we deny them the opportunity to grow. We do not have the right to make that choice.

We can never be arrogant enough to assume that we "know" (or think we know) the cognitive and functioning level of an individual with autism. Worse yet, is to equate that level with the productive value of a human being. I stand firm in my conviction that individuals with autism have much more to teach us than we have to teach them. Ego and expertise too easily get in the way of the lessons we could learn. As educators and parents we are given the privilege of being present to human beings that are rich with gifts that we cannot always see. It is our duty to work diligently to develop those gifts and expect progress. To lower our expectations is to give up on another human being. This is simply not acceptable.

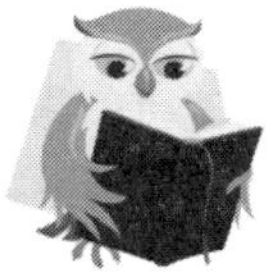

"When I was younger I was looking for this magic meaning of life. It's very simple now. Making the lives of others better, doing something of lasting value. That's the meaning of life, it's that simple."
~Temple Grandin

Appendix A: Portrait of a Student

Name of child ________________________

> **Directions:** Each year the parent or the teacher (preferably both) list information specific and significant to that child. This is an informal record or "snapshot" of the child's autism at that time. Use the information from this book, the IEP, and observations to create a portrait of your child.

What are the student's talents and strengths?

How does the student express his/her thoughts, feelings and requests? Using spoken language or augmentative communication? Describe.

What does the student understand in terms of what he/she hears and reads? Does his/her response match what you believe is understood?
Examples: being able to follow directions, understand a story, and understand figurative language and so on.

What strategies/tools have helped improve expressive and receptive language?

Does the student show any hyper-or hypo-reactivity to sensory input or unusual interest in sensory aspects of environment? Describe. (I.e. Response to pain, touch, cold, pressure, textures and so on)

What strategies or tools have been useful in helping the student to regulate sensory issues and maintain self -control?

In what independent leisure activities does the student engage (at home and at school)? I.e. Given free time what might the student choose to do?

What concerns do you have for the student's social development? What goals do you feel are important in terms of developing social communication skills?

What strategies or tools have been useful in developing social skills?

What routines, rituals, or behaviour does the student demonstrate or require consistently?

With what topics, objects or activities does the student show an intense interest? How often do these change?

What strategies or tools have been useful in incorporating his/her interests in the classroom and in individual programming?

What activities, situations or people cause an increase in anxiety in the student?

How does the student typically cope with anxiety? What signs might we see that anxiety is increasing?

What tangible objects, interests or preferred activities motivate the student?

Which strategies have been effective in easing transitions for this student? What is not effective?

What skills or tasks is the student able to do independently (even for a few minutes)?

What duration of time is the student likely to work on a task independently? Identify the task.

What functional life skills is the student able to carry out independently?

Examples:

- Self- care skills (e.g. toileting, dressing, washing/bathing, tooth brushing, eating, using Kleenex, menstrual hygiene, applying deodorant)
- Household chores (e.g., putting possessions away, setting table, loading/unloading dishwasher, sweeping)
- Personal Safety
- Public Transportation

What safety issues might pose a problem for the student? (I.e. flight risk, leaving with strangers, water, fire alarms, electricity and so on)

Describe student's gross motor skills and fine motor skills. Large muscle movements (jumping, running, balancing, skipping etc...**Fine motor skills**: printing, handwriting, painting, coloring, cutting skills etc...

What academic tasks seem to be more difficult for the student? Which are less troubling?

What components or aspects of the tasks or subject do you feel are the most challenging for the student? (I.e. Planning, organizing, computing, brainstorming, inferring, recording, attending, shifting attention, memory)

What self- advocacy skills does the student demonstrate?

What would you like to see the student be able to do in terms of self- advocacy?

What instructional strategies and approaches do you feel, have been ineffective for the student in the past?

What tasks, routines, habits or objects are a constant challenge at home or a source of tension around the house? Or is there anything specific or pressing that you would like your child to practice?

What are the student's hopes and dreams for the future?

What are the student's parents hopes and dreams for his/her future?

Concerns and questions:

Appendix B Staying on Track During an IEP Meeting

The following is a checklist of issues and needs that must be discussed and documented during the IEP meeting:

Discussion and goal setting for the following areas: (Specific, measurable, active, realistic and bound by time)	**Yes**	**No**	**Comments/Notes**
Discussion of and documentation of strengths and needs			
Identified areas of interest that will be utilized in teaching new and difficult concepts			
Discussion of assessments and reports that pertain to the student's current level of performance and learning styles.			
Discussion and documentation of how autism affects the student's ability to participate in the regular curriculum.			
Identify general curriculum modifications in specific subject areas			
Identify necessary accommodations needed to access curriculum			
Identified needs in social interactions, social skills and social language			
Identified needs in cognitive patterns (executive function, information processing, critical thinking, memory)			
Identified needs in sensory regulation (sensory diet and environmental issues)			
Identified patterns of behaviour or activities that are restricted, repetitive, or stereotypic			
Identified needs in emotional development and self- regulation			
Identified needs or accommodations in auditory processing			
Identified needs in self -care and adaptive functioning			
Identified needs in gross and/or fine motor skills			

Are the student's goals clear on *what* student will do, *how*, *where* and *when* he/she will do it?			
Methods of assessment and evaluation of goals and objectives.			
Are the educational aids and equipment (such as books on tape, modified seating, computer programs, sensory tools, access to an educational assistant and services (such as speech therapy, special day class, resource) to be provided clearly documented in the IEP?			
Identified effective teaching strategies (consider Applied Behaviour Analysis methods)			
Transportation needs noted?			
Signatures of all present?			
Copy of IEP to parent and each member			

Appendix C: Staying on Track During a Transition Plan Meeting

Transition Planning	Yes	No	Comments/Notes
Persons that are directly responsible for providing transition services were in attendance			
Student and family were in attendance			
Instructional goals, including requirements to complete certain classes to succeed in the general curriculum and to gain needed skills			
Related services to help the student achieve goals Identify the accommodations, supports, or related services that the student needs in their present education in order to meet their future transition goal			
The instruction, activities and the course of study directly relate to how the student is functioning and what he/she wants to do after high school - academic - vocational - adult living skills - self-advocacy and self-awareness			
Employment-related activities such as co-operative work placements, career exploration and supportive employment?			
Daily living skills (meal preparation, laundry, hygiene, shopping and money management			
Transportation and mobility issues (including related skills such as taking a bus, reading a schedule etc...)			
Interagency responsibilities or any needed services (Community living, social work, counseling etc...)			

Plan reflects the student's interests, hobbies and preferences			
Plan reflects the student's weaknesses based on Autism			
A vocational assessment which provides practical information about job or career interests A great website is: http://www.transitioncoalition.org			
Transition services and activities aimed at leisure activities and community involvement			
Post school financial options and support; begin the application process			
Post school housing options; begin the application process			
Transition services aimed at postsecondary education (Include information on admission requirements, academic support)			
Transition services that aimed at vocational training			
Transition services that are aimed at integrated employment (including supported employment)			
Transition services that are aimed at independent living			
Transition services that are aimed at continuing adult education			
Provide for planning follow-up or follow-along support once the student develops independence in a transition activity or once he graduates			
Notification of transfer of transition rights at age 22			

Appendix D <u>Examples of Charts for Tracking Skill Development</u>

Data should be recorded at least once a week for each objective (everyday may be necessary for some skills). When recording data for new skills it is important to record whether or not a prompt was used (P) or how many times out of a specific number of trials the student was successful (e.g. 4 out of 5). Anecdotal notes are also helpful because skills acquisition never seems as clear cut as we would like it to be. This is particularly true for individuals with autism. The more information that can be recorded is beneficial for program planning because if not written down, our teaching becomes too "hit and miss." Self -monitoring is also an excellent way to increase student engagement in learning.

Student form for self -monitoring

Goal: When the beep sound is heard, I will be on task (i.e., eyes focused on the teacher or on my work) at least 75% during math class (30 minute).

Using a digital beeper that is set to buzz every 5 minutes

Objective:	**Monday**	**Tuesday**	**Wednesday**	**Thursday**	**Friday**
Beep 1	☺	☺	☺	☺	
Beep 2		☺	☺	☺	☺
Beep 3	☺	☺	☺	☺	☺
Beep 4		☺	☺		
Beep 5					
Beep 6	☺	☺	☺	☺	☺
Total	50%	83%	83%	66%	50%

Goal: I am prepared for each class and engaged in the discussion at least 90% of the time for each subject this semester.

	Monday	**Tuesday**	**Wednesday**	**Thursday**	**Friday**
Class 1	☑ Materials ready ☑Homework complete ☑ Handed in ☑ Participated in discussion at least one time	☑ Materials ready ☑Homework complete ☑ Handed in ☑ Participated in discussion at least one time	☑ Materials ready ☑Homework complete ☑ Handed in ☑ Participated in discussion at least one time	☑ Materials ready ☑Homework complete ☑ Handed in ☑ Participated in discussion at least one time	☑ Materials ready ☑Homework complete ☑ Handed in ☑ Participated in discussion at least one time
Class 2	☑ Materials ready ☑Homework complete ☑ Handed in ☑ Participated in discussion at least one time	☑ Materials ready ☑Homework complete ☑ Handed in ☑ Participated in discussion at least one time	☑ Materials ready ☑Homework complete ☑ Handed in ☑ Participated in discussion at least one time	☑ Materials ready ☑Homework complete ☑ Handed in ☑ Participated in discussion at least one time	☑ Materials ready ☑Homework complete ☑ Handed in ☑ Participated in discussion at least one time

Appendix E: Sample Functional Behaviour Analysis

When analyzing behaviour it is essential that the behaviour be described objectively; free of any assumptions about why it happened. It is also important to note any setting events (situations or experiences that may be happening in the student's life both in and out of school that could impact on the behaviour of the student (e.g. divorce, death, illness, parents are away etc...)

Date and Time	**Antecedent What happened immediately before the behaviour?**	**Specific Behaviour Observed Describe it so that it can be acted out exactly (objectively)**	**People involved in the task or activity**	**Consequence What did others do or say during or after the behaviour? What happened?**	**Possible Function**
Sept. 23 9:40 a.m.	Teacher announces "Computer time is over" Educational Assistant moves towards computer and says, "Bob, computer is finished."	Yells "No!" Holds computer mouse in hand Remains seated, focused on screen Legs wrapped around chair legs	Teacher EA 15 students	Teacher gives a verbal reminder, "Computer time is over. Please line up."	Sensory input? Avoidance of transition?
	Teacher counts to 10 and verbally threatens loss of computer privileges for remainder of day	Student yells, "NO!" loudly Kicks the table leg 4 or 5 times with left foot Remains seated and focused on screen	Teacher EA	Teacher leaves room with 15 students	Sensory input? Or wants more time on computer? Avoidance of transition?
	EA turns off computer screen and stands beside student	Student pounds fist on table Stands up, pushes chair back and throws computer mouse across the room	EA	EA calls for assistance	Escape?

The data above will hopefully indicate to staff that the student's behaviour communicated a need/want to stay on the computer for some reason which we may not know at this point. The point to keep in mind is that our job is to **determine what needs to happen, rather than, what needs to stop**. The use of a visual warning (Time Timer™), and a First/Then schedule (or a numbered list of tasks) might have prevented the behaviour. Rather than assuming that the student is simply "non- compliant," our data shows a lack of transition support by staff as a possible cause of the behaviour. Staff needed to understand the rigid thinking patterns of individuals with autism and implement antecedent strategies.

Appendix F: What Motivates the Student?

Students with autism are sometimes more difficult to motivate. They are not always inspired by usual forms of motivation. It is essential to find out (with the help of a parent) what motivates the individual. The following is an informal inventory that a teacher could use to determine useful reinforcers for programming.

Item/Activity	Highly rewarding	Somewhat rewarding	Not going to do the job!
Social praise ("Good job!")			
Physical praise (high five or a handshake)			
Written praise (a note home)			
Sensory reward (Brushing, squeeze, vibrating chair etc...)			
Food (specify a few)			
Stickers			
Toys (specify)			
Small badges or awards			
Free time in classroom			
Time in the gymnasium			
A visit to a special person in the school (custodian or the principal)			
Walk outside			
Time to draw			
Time to listen to music			
Lego or other building game			

Item/Activity	Highly rewarding	Somewhat rewarding	Not going to do the job!
Going to the library			
Time in a quiet spot (classroom tent)			
Movie time (this can be as little as 5 minutes!)			
Popcorn party			
Trampoline			
Bubble blowing			
Sand table or water table			
Book on tape			
Free reading time			
Sit with a buddy			
Classroom job			
Play with a class pet			
Computer/ipad time			
Eat lunch out of the classroom			
Collect a desired item from a set (cards)			
Field trip to a restaurant or favorite store			
Game time			
Extra recess time			

Appendix G: Checking In: A Checklist for Setting up a Classroom for a Student with Autism Spectrum Disorder

Teaching students with autism involves some extra thinking that educators don't necessarily have to consider for more typical students. However, the points below are very appropriate for any student with special needs or learning differences. The checklist is far from exhaustive but it does provide a sense of what aspects of classroom set –up and organization that need attention for students with autism.

Physical Organization		
Is the student's desk in a place where he will feel safe? (Anyone behind him? Is she on a perimeter of the room?)		
Are the walls too distracting? Use only instructional materials. Is an area available for working alone, free from people and distractions?		
Has a "safe spot" been identified where student can go when needed? Not for punishment!		
Are clear pathways set up for purposeful movement? Observe the student's movement through the class to determine if areas need to be rearranged.		
Is the locker in a place that is easily monitored by adults or a peer buddy?		
Will the student know where to put finished work? And what to do when work is done?		
Are the surfaces that the student accesses clear? Book shelves, desk top, locker, activity centers?		
Are the instructions or expectations for activity centers clearly marked? Where are the materials for the task? Where do materials go when task is complete? Are the materials in the order that they will be used?		
Does the setup of the classroom and the materials foster independence? (Or will the student need to depend on someone else to find materials and move from one activity to the next)		

Teaching and Learning Materials		
Is a personal visual schedule on or near the student's desk?		
Does the schedule clearly indicate what happens next? Where?		
Do the visual symbols reflect the developmental level of the child? (Symbols need to "grow" with the student: objects, photos, pictures, line drawings/symbols and then written text) i.e. a high		

functioning student will probably be using the written word with some pictures)		
Are the student's materials color coded or visually organized for each subject? (i.e. a blue dot on each material needed for math)		
Are materials arranged in a way that helps the student organize his thinking? (trays in the desk, file folders, books in sequence for the order of the daily instruction) "Everything in its place"		
Does the locker contain a copy of the class schedule, materials needed and map of the school?		
Are worksheets uncluttered? Ample space for largely printed answers?		
Are instructions clear and to the point? If not, cover them and rewrite with precise steps.		
Is the student able to respond using his learning style? (Oral, matching, pointing, written, computer etc...)		
Is there a balance between seatwork and tasks that involve hands on and kinesthetic activity?		
Does the setup of some of the tasks and activities foster independence? (Will the student be able to experience a level of independence on some tasks in order to develop self -esteem and a "can do" attitude?)		
Are coping strategies readily available to the student; sensory tools, relaxation booklets, social scripts etc...		
Has a motivational assessment been done to determine what can be used to motivate the student? (Tangible, sensory, food, social rewards)		
Is the curriculum for this student designed to reflect the nature of autism? Have the "autism goals" been set? (Social, communication, anxiety, sensory and behavioural programs)		

Assessment		**Comments**
Have formal tests been done and recommendations recorded? (Psycho-Educational tests, the Assessment of Basic Language and Learning Skills (the ABLLS)		
Have informal assessments been conducted to determine baseline data? (data collected before intervention or teaching strategies are employed) Informal assessments could be observation, interview, behavioural checklists, and curriculum-based assessments.		

Are strategies in place to collect data on social, communication, academic and possibly behaviour?		
Does the assessment match the learning style of the student? Does it contain visual, auditory, and/or kinesthetic components?		
Is the student able to respond using his strongest learning style or ability? (matching, oral, pointing, choosing, yes/no)		
Is the time of day the most productive for the student? (As the day wears on these students are exhausted from the social/emotional demands of the day)		
Is the location or setting the most productive for the student? (Assessing a student while he is surrounded by other people may not be the most reflective of his abilities due to the stress of the environment)		
Are the instructions given in a way that the student understands? (Pairing visual and auditory is often the most effective)		
Is assessment done over a series of days or times of day in order to get a fair reflection of what capabilities the student has?		

Appendix H: People with Autism that Inspire Us

Dr. Temple Grandin, Ph.D. food animal handling systems designer, author and public speaker www.templegrandin.com (see References for list of books and interviews)

Donna Williams, author of, *Nobody Nowhere: The Extraordinary Autobiography of an Autistic* (1992) and *Somebody Somewhere: Breaking Free from the World of Autism* (1993) and many more

Dr. Stephen Shore, author of *Beyond the Wall: Personal Experiences with Autism and Asperger Syndrome* and editor of *Ask and Tell: Self-Advocacy and Disclosure for People on the Autism Spectrum;* www.autismasperger.net

Luke Jackson, author of, *Freaks, Geeks and Asperger Sydrome: A User Guide to Adolescences* (2002)

John Elder Robison, author of *Look Me in the Eye: My Life with Asperger's 2007*

Jerry and Mary Newport, author of *Your Life Is Not a Label: A Guide to Living Fully with Autism and Asperger's Syndrome for Parents, Professionals and You!* (2001) and *Autism - Asperger's and Sexuality: Puberty and Beyond* (2002) - with Mary Newport www.aspires-relationships.com (**Mary Newport** author of, *Autism - Asperger's and Sexuality: Puberty and Beyond* (2002) - with Jerry Newport)

Liane Holliday Willey, author of, *Pretending to be Normal, Asperger Syndrome in the Family, Pretending to Be Normal: Living with Asperger's Syndrome* (1999), *Asperger Syndrome in the Family: Redefining Normal* (2001), *Asperger Syndrome in Adolescence: Living with the Ups, the Downs and Things in Between*

Jasmine O'Neill, a mute autistic savant, is a poet, writer, illustrator, musician and author of *Through the Eyes of Aliens (*1999 Jessica Kingsley Publishers)

Lucy Blackman , author of *Lucy's Story: Autism and Other Adventures* (1999)

Sean Barron, author of, *There's A Boy In Here* (1992) - with Judy Barron

Carly Fleishman non-verbal author and advocate living with autism **-** http://carlysvoice.com and https://www.youtube.com/watch?v=KmDGvquzn2k

Tito Mukhopadhyay http://ngm.nationalgeographic.com/ngm/0503/feature1/online_extra.html https://www.youtube.com/watch?v=Nfiap3a7Tuo

Jenna Lumbard, non-verbal author and advocate living with autism
http://www.autismsupportnetwork.com/news/video-jenna-lumbard-non-verbal-autistic-author-98273633
http://exertyourrightoknow.blogspot.ca/2010/07/video-jenna-lumbard-non-verbal-autistic.html

Naoki Higashida, was 13 years old at the time he wrote the memoir, and nonverbal. (He is now 21 years old.)

Daniel Tammet, author (2006) Born on a Blue Day: A Memoir. New York: Thorndike Press

Appendix J: Assistive Technology Selection and Implementation Guide

Dr. Todd Cunningham is a registered as a psychologist in Ontario (Canada). The following online resource for Assistive Technology and Academic Support Services for students is based on his study and clinical work. The Assistive Technology Tool Selection Protocol provides a comprehensive model for guiding a clinician or educator to identify the appropriate technology to support the specific learning needs a student may have. It is highly recommended that the reader visit Dr. Cunningham's website at www.learndifferent.org in order to see the full instructions and links to using the Assistive Technology Selection and Implementation Guide. It is an excellent tool to guide the important decisions being made around using technology to "circumvent a skill that is absent or impaired."

The process consists of 4 steps. The information form each of these steps can be recorded on the work page Assistive Technology Selection and Implementation Guide below.

1. Use the SETT framework to identify to identify ecological variables (Zabala, 2000; Virtual Center of Excellence, 2000). SETT stands for a) Student, b) Environment, c) Task, and d) Tool.

2. Once SETT variables have been considered, use the Assistive Technology Map below to identify the assistive technology tool. To do, first identify the main domain the student is having a difficulty with (oral language, reading, writing, season/motor, organization, or math). Next, identify the specific academic skill that is interfering. For example, reading is comprised of decoding/fluency, comprehension, and reading vocabulary. The final step will be the identifying of the appropriate assistive technology tool.

3. Once you have identified the assistive technology tool, then learn more about the tool in the Assistive Technology Tool List from the website LearnDifferent.org

4. After deciding the appropriate assistive technology tool, next choose the program. Look through the assistive technology program software and the equipment list to find a suitable program. When making this decision, take back into consideration the SETT variables.

SETT FRAMEWORK

- S = Student
- E = Environment
- T = the Task
- T = the Tools

The Student

- What does the student need to do?
- What are the student's current abilities?
- What are the student's special needs?
- Can the student articulate what their strengths and weaknesses are?

The Environments

- What are the instructional and physical arrangements?
- Are there special concerns?
- What materials and equipment are currently available in the environment?
- What supports are available to the student and the people working with the student on a daily basis?

- How are the attitudes and expectations of the people in the environment likely to affect the student's performance?

Task:

- What is everyone else doing in the classroom?
- What are the critical elements of the activities?
- Based on the students learning profile, what are the barriers that are preventing them from doing the activities?

Tool:

- Are systems of assistive technology tools and strategies required for a student with these needs and abilities to do these tasks in these environments?
- What no tech, low tech, and high tech options should be considered for inclusion in an assistive technology system for a student with these needs and abilities doing these tasks in these environments?
- How might the student's special needs be accommodated without changing the critical elements of the activities?
- Will modifications of the critical elements of the activities be necessary to promote the student's participation?
- What strategies might be used to increase student performance?
- How might the student try out the proposed system of tools in the environments which they will be used?

All Students Learn

Feel Safe
+ Motivated
+ KNOW THEIR STRENGTHS
+ Compensatory & Remediation
+ Support Network

= Their GOALS

Dr. Todd Cunningham, 2008

Cunningham, T. (2008) http://pogoforsurvivors.files.wordpress.com/2014/01/workshop-e_-a-leg-up-assistive-technology.pdf

Retrieved with permission from www.learndifferent.org on August 1, 2014

SETT based on work by Joy Smiley Zabala Setting the Stage for Success: Building Success Through Effective Selection and Use of Assistive Technology Systems (2000)

http://www.ldonline.org/article/Setting_the_Stage_for_Success%3A__Building_Success_Through_Effective__Selection_and_Use_of__Assistive_Technology_Systems?theme=prin

Assistive Technology Selection and Implementation Guide

Student Information		
Student Name	Grade	Age
School	Date	AT Plan Review Date

Staff Contact (Individual assigned to assess and implement the plan)

About the Student (IEP, Assessment Data)	
Diagnosis:	
Cognitive Profile	
Strengths	Challenges
Academic Profile	
Strengths	Challenges

Environment Considerations

Task:			
Academic Tasks	Demands of task	What are the skills being taught or tested?	What skills are needed to show knowledge of skill being taught or tested? Which skills need to be supported?

Assistive Technology Selection:			
Academic Skill	Assistive Technology Tool	Assistive Technology Product	Environmental Considerations

Training			
Training Needs	Trainer	Dates & Times	Follow Up

Assistive Technology Product Provider	
Equipment & Software to be used	Sources (e.g. School | S.E.A. | Home | Need to Purchase | Other)

Monitoring/Evaluation		
Goals	Instructional Strategy (How you will teach student to use equipment and/or how to achieve goals?)	Recording System & Frequency (e.g., task analysis recording system; score "+" or "-" on the data recoding sheet)

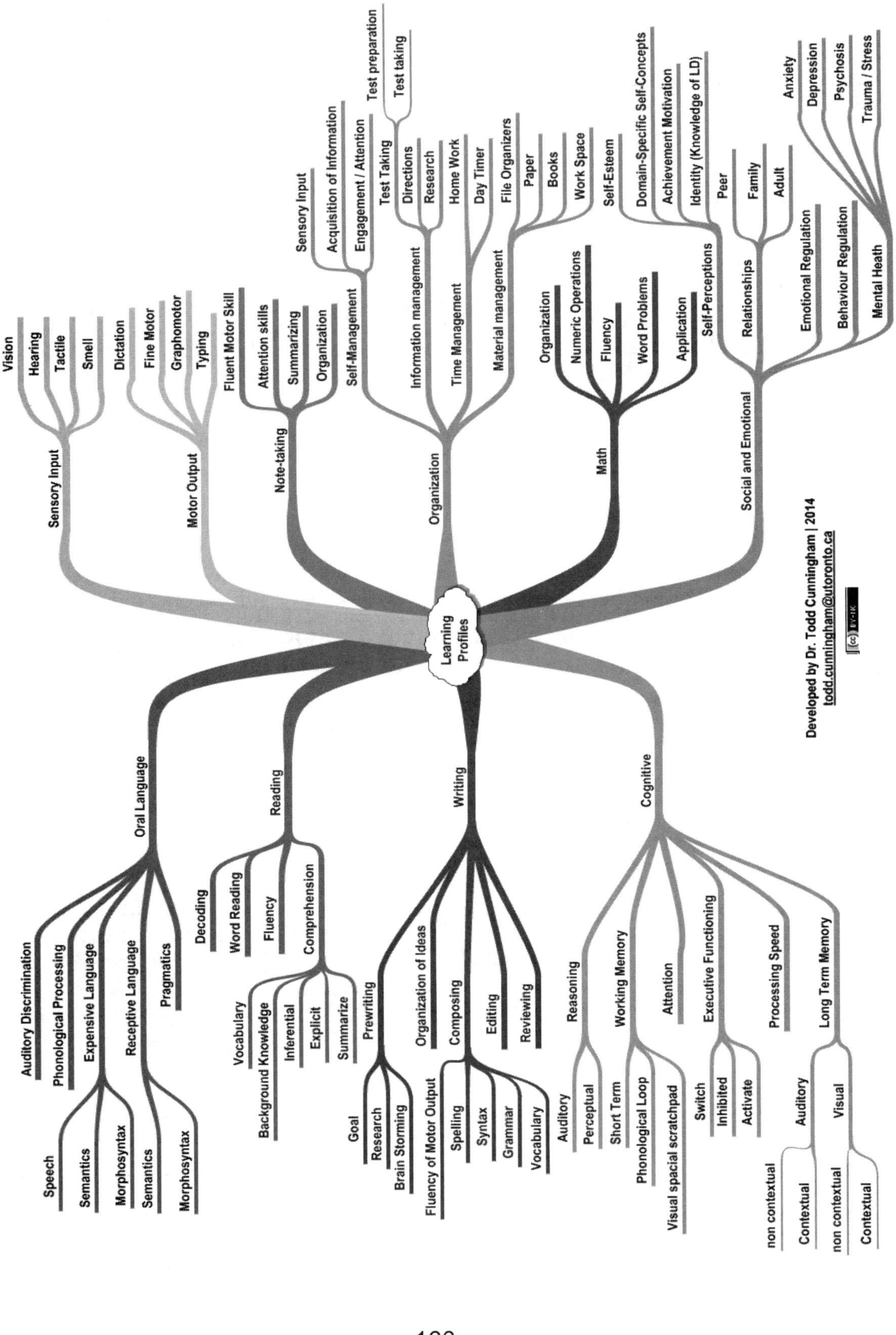

Learning Profiles
Sensory Input
Vision
Hearing
Tactile
Smell
Motor Output
Dictation
Fine Motor
Graphomotor
Typing
Note-taking
Fluent Motor Skill
Attention skills
Summarizing
Organization
Organization
Self-Management
Sensory Input
Acquisition of Information
Engagement / Attention
Test Taking
Test preparation
Test taking
Information management
Directions
Research
Home Work
Time Management
Day Timer
Material management
File Organizers
Paper
Books
Work Space
Math
Organization
Numeric Operations
Fluency
Word Problems
Application
Social and Emotional
Self-Perceptions
Self-Esteem
Domain-Specific Self-Concepts
Achievement Motivation
Identity (Knowledge of LD)
Relationships
Peer
Family
Adult
Emotional Regulation
Behaviour Regulation
Mental Heath
Anxiety
Depression
Psychosis
Trauma / Stress
Oral Language
Auditory Discrimination
Phonological Processing
Expensive Language
Speech
Semantics
Morphosyntax
Receptive Language
Semantics
Morphosyntax
Pragmatics
Reading
Decoding
Word Reading
Fluency
Comprehension
Vocabulary
Background Knowledge
Inferential
Explicit
Summarize
Writing
Prewriting
Goal
Research
Brain Storming
Organization of Ideas
Composing
Fluency of Motor Output
Spelling
Syntax
Grammar
Vocabulary
Editing
Reviewing
Cognitive
Reasoning
Auditory
Perceptual
Working Memory
Short Term
Phonological Loop
Visual spacial scratchpad
Attention
Executive Functioning
Switch
Inhibited
Activate
Processing Speed
Long Term Memory
Auditory
non contextual
Contextual
Visual
non contextual
Contextual
Developed by Dr. Todd Cunningham | 2014
todd.cunningham@utoronto.ca
BY-NC

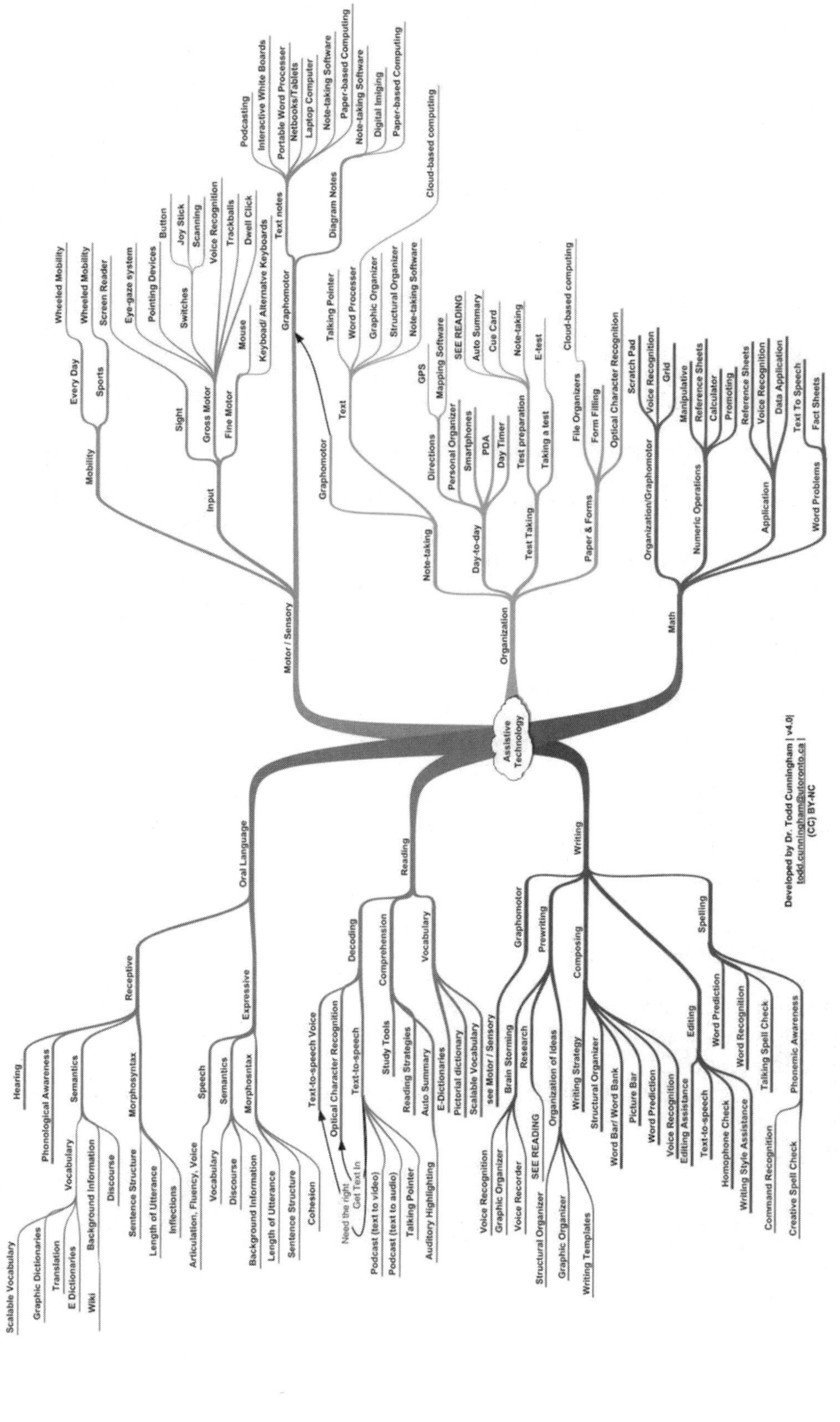
Assistive Technology
Motor / Sensory
Mobility
Every Day
Wheeled Mobility
Sports
Wheeled Mobility
Screen Reader
Input
Sight
Gross Motor
Fine Motor
Eye-gaze system
Pointing Devices
Switches
Button
Joy Stick
Scanning
Voice Recognition
Trackballs
Dwell Click
Mouse
Keyboad/ Alternatve Keyboards
Graphomotor
Text notes
Podcasting
Interactive White Boards
Portable Word Processer
Netbooks/Tablets
Laptop Computer
Note-taking Software
Paper-based Computing
Diagram Notes
Note-taking Software
Digital Imaging
Paper-based Computing
Cloud-based computing
Organization
Note-taking
Graphomotor
Text
Talking Pointer
Word Processer
Graphic Organizer
Structural Organizer
Note-taking Software
Day-to-day
Directions
GPS
Mapping Software
Personal Organizer
Smartphones
PDA
Day Timer
Test Taking
Test preparation
SEE READING
Auto Summary
Cue Card
Note-taking
Taking a test
E-test
Paper & Forms
File Organizers
Form Filling
Optical Character Recognition
Cloud-based computing
Math
Organization/Graphomotor
Scratch Pad
Voice Recognition
Grid
Numeric Operations
Manipulative
Reference Sheets
Calculator
Promoting
Application
Reference Sheets
Voice Recognition
Data Application
Word Problems
Text To Speech
Fact Sheets
Oral Language
Receptive
Hearing
Phonological Awareness
Semantics
Vocabulary
Scalable Vocabulary
Graphic Dictionaries
Translation
E Dictionaries
Wiki
Background Information
Discourse
Morphosyntax
Sentence Structure
Length of Utterance
Inflections
Expressive
Speech
Articulation, Fluency, Voice
Semantics
Vocabulary
Discourse
Background Information
Morphosntax
Length of Utterance
Sentence Structure
Cohesion
Reading
Decoding
Text-to-speech Voice
Optical Character Recognition
Text-to-speech
Need the right
Get Text In
Podcast (text to video)
Podcast (text to audio)
Talking Pointer
Auditory Highlighting
Comprehension
Study Tools
Reading Strategies
Auto Summary
Vocabulary
E-Dictionaries
Pictorial dictionary
Scalable Vocabulary
Writing
Graphomotor
see Motor / Sensory
Prewriting
Brain Storming
Voice Recognition
Graphic Organizer
Voice Recorder
Research
SEE READING
Structural Organizer
Organization of Ideas
Graphic Organizer
Writing Templates
Composing
Writing Strategy
Structural Organizer
Word Bar/ Word Bank
Picture Bar
Word Prediction
Voice Recognition
Editing Assistance
Editing
Text-to-speech
Homophone Check
Writing Style Assistance
Command Recognition
Creative Spell Check
Spelling
Word Prediction
Word Recognition
Talking Spell Check
Phonemic Awareness
Developed by Dr. Todd Cunningham | v4.0|
todd.cunningham@utoronto.ca |
(CC) BY-NC

Appendix I: Helpful Resources

Self- Awareness and Self Esteem

Peter Vemeulen, I AM Special 2: A Workbook to Help Children, Teens and Adults with Autism Spectrum Disorders to Understand Their Diagnosis, Gain Confidence and Thrive. (Jessica Kingsley, 2013)

Temple Grandin and Kate Duffy, *Developing Talents: Careers For Individuals With Asperger Syndrome And High-functioning Autism.* Updated, Expanded Edition (Autism Asperger Publishing Company, 2008)

Elaine Larson, I Am Utterly Unique: Celebrating the Strength of Children with Asperger Syndrome and High-Functioning Autism. (Autism Asperger Publishing Company, 2006).

UCSC Autism Research Program, www.psy.ucsd.edu/autism/prttraining

www.aspergeradults.ca/aspergrgrrrlz (This site is for females with Asperger's Syndrome)

http://www.ldonline.org/article/5736/ (Memory Strategies)

Ability Online http://www.abilityonline.org/ Ability Online is an incredibly supportive online community for kids, teens and young adults with all kinds of disabilities or chronic illnesses. It allows any member (child, teen or parent) to connect with others for friendship, support and information in a secure, bully-free environment where the goal is to help our members accomplish great things! Membership is free. Programs for the youth include Bully Bouncers, Friendship Builder and Transition Plus.

Model Me Kids www.modelmekids.com

TD Social Skills www.tdsocialskills.com

Michelle Garcia - Winner, Think Social! A Social Thinking Curriculum for School-Age Students. (2nd Printing) (Think Social Publishing, Inc., 2008)

Stephanie Madrigal & Michele Garcia Winner, Superflex Takes on Glassman and the Team of Unthinkables. (Think Social Publishing, 2009)

Augmentative Communication

Talking Rockets – Extremely affordable ($99)! MyVoice Inc makes RocketKeys and TalkRocket Go apps that are very easy to use! Using an iPhone or iPad, these apps give people with speech and language disabilities a voice!
http://myvoiceaac.com/2012/07/introducing-talkrocket-go-the-successor-to-myvoice/

www.pecs.com

Play

Julia Moor, *Playing, Laughing and Learning with Children on the Autism Spectrum.* (Jessica Kingsley Publishers, 2008)

Melinda Smith, *Teaching Playskills to Children with Autism Spectrum.* (DRL Books, 2001)

Jed Baker, No More Meltdowns. (Future Horizons, 2008)

Self-Regulation and Emotional Development

Tony Attwood, *Exploring Feelings: Cognitive Behaviour Therapy to Manage Anger. (Future Horizons, 2004)*

Tony Attwood, *Exploring Feelings: Cognitive Behaviour Therapy to Manage Anxiety. (Future Horizons, 2004)*

Lori Lite, *The Angry Octopus* (Stress Free Kids, 2008) Check out all of Lori's books for children. They are excellent tools for coping with stress and negative emotions. Go to www.autismaspirations.com and scroll to the link at the bottom of the first page

Leah Kutpers, Zones of Regulation. (Think Social Publishing, 2011)

Sherry Moyer, *The Eclipse Model: Teaching Self Regulation, Executive Function, Attribution, and Sensory Awareness to Students with Asperger Syndrome, High Functioning Autism, and Related Disorders.* (Autism Asperger Publishing Co., 2009)

Elisa Gagnon, *Power Cards: Using Special Interests to Motivate Children and Youth with Asperger Syndrome and Autism.* (Autism Asperger Publishing Company, 2001)

Sensory Help

Carol Kranowitz & Lucy Jane Miller, *The Out-of-Sync Child: Recognizing and Coping with Sensory Processing Disorder.* Revised Edition, (Perigree Trade, 2006)

Cognition and Executive Function

Lynn Cannon et. al., Unstuck and on Target! An Executive Function Curriculum to Improve Flexibility For Children With Autism Spectrum Disorders. (Brooks Publishing Research Edition, 2011)

Peg Dawson, & Richard Guare, Smart but Scattered: The Revolutionary "Executive Skills" Approach to Helping Kids Reach Their Potential. (The Guilford Press, 2009)

http://cft.vanderbilt.edu/guides-sub-pages/visual-thinking/

Transition Planning

Jed Baker, *Preparing for Life: The Complete Guide for Transitioning to Adulthood for Those with Autism and Asperger's Syndrome. (Future Horizons, 2006)*

http://autismnow.org/articles/best-practices-in-the-transition-from-high-school-to-adult-for-individuals-with-asd-and-other-developmental-disorders/#sthash.hZQ7vQKf.dpuf

More Good Resources

www.timetimer.com

Autism Research Institute, www.autism.com

www.cairn-site.com CAIRN: Canadian Autism Intervention Research Network

DO2LEARN - www.dotolearn.com A web site providing activities to promote independence in children and adults with special learning needs.

Temple Grandin, The Way I See It: A Personal Look at Autism and Asperger's. 2nd edition, (Future Horizons, 2011)

Ruth Aspy, & Barry Grossman, Ziggurat Model and CAPS Forms http://texasautism.com/blog/training/forms/

EIC – ASD Enhancing Instructional Contexts for Students with Autism Spectrum Disorders Juane Heflin, PhD & Kristen Hess, MA http://coeweb.gsu.edu/autism//instrument.pdf

Brenda Smith -Myles, The Hidden Curriculum: Practical Solutions for Understanding Unstated Rules in Social Situations. (Autism Asperger Publishing Company, 2004)

Peter Wright, Emotions to Advocacy. (Harbor House Law Press; 2 edition, 2006) http://www.wrightslaw.com/bks/feta2/feta2.skim.pdf

Emily Iland, Drawing a Blank: Improving Comprehension for Readers on the Autism Spectrum. (Autism Aspergers Publishing Co. 2011)

References

Aspy, R. and Grossman, B. (2008) The Ziggurat Model. Kansas: AAPC, pg. 209.

Attwood, T. (2008). The Complete Guide to Asperger's Syndrome. London: Jessica Kingsley Publishers.

Bowler, D. M., Gardiner, J. M., & Grice, S. J. (2000). Episodic memory and remembering in adults with asperger syndrome. Journal of Autism and Developmental Disorders, 30, 295–304. doi:10.1023/A: 1005575216176

Cesaroni and Garber, (1991) *Exploring the experience of autism through firsthand accounts*. Journal of Autism and Developmental Disorders, Volume 21, Number 3.

Dweck, C. Mindset: The New Psychology of Success Random House Publishing Group | December 26, 2007 |

Eltz, D. (2002, October) Bedeviled No More: Autism Linked to Rapid Brain Growth. Pittmed. http://pittmed.health.pitt.edu/Oct_2002/PITTMED_Oct2002.pdf

Franke, L. & Dunn, C. (2011) Nurturing Narratives. Kansas: Autism Aspergers Publishing Company

Gaigg, S., Bowler, D. Gardiner, J. (2014). *Episodic but not semantic order memory difficulties in autism spectrum disorder: evidence from the historical figures task*. Memory, 2014; 22(6):669-78. doi: 10.1080/09658211.2013.811256. Epub 2013 Jul 1.

Grandin, T. (1995). *Thinking in pictures and other reports from my life with autism*. New York: Doubleday.

Grandin, T. (2006) *Thinking in pictures: my life with autism. 2nd edition,* New York: Vintage Books.

Grandin, T. (2009) *How does visual thinking work in the mind of a person with autism? A personal account.* Department of Animal Sciences, Colorado State University, Fort Collins, CO

80523, USA Philosophical Transactions of the Royal Society 364, 1437-1442 Retrieved on August 1, 2014 doi: 10.1098/rstb.2008.0297

Grandin, T. & Panek, R. (2013) The Autistic Brain: Thinking Across the Spectrum. Boston: Houghton Mifflin.

Greenspan, S. (1995). *The Challenging Child: Understanding, Raising, and Enjoying the Five "Difficult" Types of Children.* Cambridge, MA: Perseus Books Group.

Herbert, D. & Burt, J. (2004) What do Students Remember? Episodic Memory and the Development of Schematization. Applied Cognitive Psychology, 18: 77–88 Published online in Wiley Inter Science (www.interscience.wiley.com) DOI: 10.1002/acp.947

Hilton. C. L., Zhang, Y., White, M. R., Klohr, & C.L., Constantino, J.(2012) Motor impairment in sibling pairs concordant and discordant for autism spectrum disorders. *Autism.*

Higashida, N. (2013). *The Reason I Jump: The Inner Voice of a Thirteen-Year-Old Boy with Autism.* Knopf Canada.

Just, M., Cherkassky,V..Timothy A. Keller1, Rajesh K. Kana1 and Nancy J. Minshew (2007) Functional and Anatomical Cortical Underconnectivity in Autism: Evidence from an fMRI Study of an Executive Function Task and Corpus Callosum Morphometry.

Kana, R.K., Keller, T.A., Cherkassky, V.L., Minshew, N.J, & Just, M.A. (2006). Sentence comprehension in autism: Thinking in pictures with decreased functional connectivity. *Brain, 129,* 2484–2493.

Kenworthy, L., Gutermuth Anthony, L.,Alexander K.C., Adler Werner, M., Cannon, L. & Greenman, L. (2014) Solving Executive Function Challenges: Simple Ways to Get Kids with Autism Unstuck & on Target. Baltimore: Brooks Publishing Co.

Kluth, P. (2008). Just Give Him the Whale: 20 Ways to Use Fascinations, Areas of Expertise, and Strengths to Support Students with Autism. Baltimore: Brooks Publishing.

Kohler, P. D., & Field, S. (2003). Transition-focused education: Foundation for the future. Journal of Special Education, 37(3), 174-183.

Koshino, H., Carpenter, P. A., Minshew, N. J., Cherkassky, V. L., Keller, T. A., & Just, M. A. (2005). Functional connectivity in an fMRI working memory task with high-functioning autism. Neuroimage, 24, 810–821.

MacDonald, M., Lord, C., & Ulrich, D. A. (2014) Motor Skills and Calibrated Autism Severity in Young Children with Autism Spectrum Disorder. *Adapted Physical Activity Quarterly*, (31) 2 DOI: 10.1123/apaq.2013-0068

Mason, R.A., Williams, D.L., Kana, R.K., Minshew, N. J., & Just, M. A. (2008). Theory of mind disruption and recruitment of the right hemisphere during narrative comprehension in autism. *Neuropsychologia, 46,* 269–280.

Minshew, N. J., Meyer, J. & Goldstein, G. 2002. Abstract reasoning in autism--a disassociation between concept formation and concept identification. Neuropsychology 16, 327-334. (doi:10.1037/0894-4105.16.3.327)

Minshew, N.J., & Williams, D.L. (2007). The new neurobiology of autism: Cortex, connectivity, and neuronal organization. *Archives of Neurology, 64,* 945–950. (doi:10.1001/archneur.64.7.945)

Minshew, N. (2006) *Children with Autism Found to Have Specific Memory Problems that May Underlie Aspects of Disorder. Retrieved* http://www.apa.org/news/press/releases/2006/01/autism.aspx

Newport, J., Newport, M. & Dodd, J. (2007) *Mozart and the Whale: An Asperger's Love Story.* New York: Touchstone.

Skoyles, J. R. (2011). *Autism, Context/Non-context Information Processing and Atypical Development.* Autism Research and Treatment Article ID 681627, http://dx.doi.org/10.1155/2011/681627

Tammet, D. (2006) Born on a Blue Day: A Memoir. New York: Thorndike Press.

Test, D. W., Fowler, C. H., Richter, S. M., White, J., Mazzotti, V., Walker, A. R., et al. (2009). Evidence-based practices in secondary transition. Career Development for Exceptional Individuals, 32(2), 115-128.

Vermeulen, P. (2012) Autism as Context Blindness. Kansas: Autism Aspergers Publishing Company.

Williams, D. L., Goldstein, G., & Minshew, N. J. (2006). Neuropsychologic Functioning in Children with Autism: Further Evidence for Disordered Complex Information Processing. Child Neuropsychology, 12, 279 - 298

Williams, D. L. & Minshew, N. J. (2010). How the Brain Thinks in Autism: Implications for Language Intervention. The ASHA Leader.

Williams, D., Goldstein, G., & Minshew, N. J., (2006) The Profile of Memory Function in Children with Autism, *Neuropsychology*, Vol. 20, No. 1.

Online References

Attwood, T. & Gray, C. (199). Discovery of "Aspie" Criteria Retrieved with permission at http://www.tonyattwood.com.au/index.htm, "Tony's Publications"

Cunningham, T. (2011) Assistive Technology Implementation Guide. www.learndifferent.org
Email: todd.cunningham@utoronto.ca Consultation Contact Information
Phone: 416.970.3433

DSM – V Diagnostic Criteria, Autism Speaks, retrieved on January 15, 2014 from http://www.autismspeaks.org/what-autism/diagnosis/dsm-5-diagnostic-criteria

Fleischmann, Carly: http://carlysvoice.com/ and https://www.youtube.com/watch?v=KmDGvquzn2k

Graham, J. & Wright, P. *2004 IDEA Transition Checklist.* http://www.wrightslaw.com/info/trans.plan.graham.htm

Grandin, T. (2014) *Social Problems: Understanding Emotions and Developing Talents* Retrieved on August 19, 2014 http://www.iidc.indiana.edu

Lumbard, Jenna, http://www.autismsupportnetwork.com/news/video-jenna-lumbard-non-verbal-autistic-author-98273633#ixzz3Bj1EtcaF

Mukhopadhyay, Tito, http://ngm.nationalgeographic.com/ngm/0503/feature1/online_extra.html https://www.youtube.com/watch?v=Nfiap3a7Tuo

National Institute on Deafness and Other Communication Disorders. NIH Workshop on Nonverbal School-Aged Children with Autism. April, 2010. http://www.nidcd.nih.gov/funding/programs/10autism/pages/detail.aspx

The National Autistic Society, www.nas.org.uk

The Newsletter of Achievers Unlimited, Inc., Fields of Vision, Volume 1, Number 6 (March 1996).

"Our Aspirations are Our Possibilities"

Dr. Samuel Johnson

Visit Autism Aspirations
www.autismaspirations.com
krumins@autismaspirations.com